MEDICALIZING DIFFERENCE

CRITICAL INTERVENTIONS IN THE MEDICAL AND HEALTH HUMANITIES

Series Editors

Stuart Murray, Corinne Saunders, Sowon Park and Angela Woods

Critical Interventions in the Medical and Health Humanities promotes a broad range of scholarly work across the Medical and Health Humanities, including both larger-scale intellectual projects and argument-led provocations, to present new field-defining, interdisciplinary research into health and human experience.

Titles in the Series

Abortion Ecologies in Southern African Fiction, Caitlin E. Stobie
COVID-19 and Shame, Fred Cooper, Luna Dolezal and Arthur Rose
Cocaine, Literature, and Culture, 1876-1930, Douglas R.J. Small
Medical Humanities and Disability Studies, Stuart Murray
Relating Suicide, Anne Whitehead

Forthcoming Titles

Autism and the Empathy Epidemic, Janet Harbold
Reproductive Health, Literature, and Print Culture, 1650–1800, Ashleigh Blackwood

MEDICALIZING DIFFERENCE

The Eighteenth-Century Construction of the "Hermaphrodite"

STEPHANIE M. HILGER

BLOOMSBURY ACADEMIC
LONDON • NEW YORK • OXFORD • NEW DELHI • SYDNEY

BLOOMSBURY ACADEMIC
Bloomsbury Publishing Plc
50 Bedford Square, London, WC1B 3DP, UK
1385 Broadway, New York, NY 10018, USA
29 Earlsfort Terrace, Dublin 2, Ireland

First published in Great Britain 2024

Cover design: Rebecca Heselton
Series design by Rebecca Heselton
Cover image © Mertrud, Antoine (and Jacques-Fabien Gautier d'Agoty). *Hermaphrodite, Dissertation au sujet de la fameuse hermaphrodite qui a paru aux yeux du public depuis environ trois mois*. Paris: Berryer, 1749.

A catalogue record for this book is available from the British Library.

Library of Congress Cataloging-in-Publication Data
Names: Hilger, Stephanie M. (Stephanie Mathilde), author.
Title: Medicalizing difference : the eighteenth-century construction of the 'hermaphrodite' / Stephanie M. Hilger, University of Illinois Urbana-Champaign, USA.
Description: London, UK ; New York, NY : Bloomsbury Academic, 2024. |
Series: Critical interventions in the medical and health humanities |
Includes bibliographical references and index.
Identifiers: LCCN 2024010982 (print) | LCCN 2024010983 (ebook) |
ISBN 9781350374928 (hardback) | ISBN 9781350374966 (paperback) |
ISBN 9781350374935 (pdf) | ISBN 9781350374942 (ebook)
Subjects: LCSH: Intersexuality–History–18th century. | Intersex people–History–18th century. | Intersexuality–Social aspects–History–18th century. | Gender nonconformity–History–18th century. | Gender-nonconforming people–History–18th century. | Gender nonconformity–Social aspects–History–18th century.
Classification: LCC RC883 .H54 2024 (print) | LCC RC883 (ebook) |
DDC 616.6/94–dc23/eng/20240627
LC record available at https://lccn.loc.gov/2024010982
LC ebook record available at https://lccn.loc.gov/2024010983

ISBN: HB: 978-1-3503-7492-8
ePDF: 978-1-3503-7493-5
eBook: 978-1-3503-7494-2

Series: Critical Interventions in the Medical and Health Humanities

Typeset by Newgen KnowledgeWorks Pvt. Ltd., Chennai, India

CONTENTS

PREFACE AND ACKNOWLEDGMENTS

Writing a preface is always a reflective task as one converses with an earlier version of oneself. When I started working on this manuscript, I did not know that the research related to it would lead me on a path toward the Medical/Health Humanities, not only in my scholarship and teaching but also at an institutional level. It began with the creation of a Medical Humanities research group at my university's Humanities Research Institute and developed into a broader initiative that sought to engage the university's newly created College of Medicine through a lecture series, a curricular initiative, and an outreach component. My involvement in the college deepened over the years and, as I am writing this preface, I am teaching an elective on the topic of "Medicine in Literature" for medical students.

In addition to having been cross-fertilized by my foray into the field of Health Humanities, *Medicalizing Difference* is deeply rooted in my previous research and teaching on eighteenth-century literature and culture, especially with respect to questions of gender and sexuality. My book, *Gender and Genre: German Women Write the French Revolution* (2014), discussed, among other things, protagonists who cross-dressed as soldiers to participate in the French Revolutionary Wars. Additionally, for many years, I had been teaching a literature course highlighting gender and sexuality. One of the key texts in that course was the nineteenth-century memoir of Herculine Barbin, a so-called "hermaphrodite," whose life story was recovered and edited by Michel Foucault in the 1970s. My research and teaching converged in my work on individuals with nonstandard sexual anatomies in the eighteenth century and their intersections with different types of nonbinary gender expression.

My research for this book has been generously supported by the University of Illinois, in the form of fellowships from the Illinois Program for Research in the Humanities (now the Humanities Research Institute) and the Center for Advanced Study. Most consequential might have been the Faculty Fellowship for Study in a Second Discipline from the College of Liberal Arts and Sciences, which allowed me to audit courses in the medical school. In my quest to understand individuals with nonstandard sexual anatomy, called "hermaphrodites" in the eighteenth century, I attended a course on embryology. The course outlined the development, in utero, of all major organ systems. When I entered the lecture hall, I stepped into a world that was both alien and fascinating to me. Having been trained entirely in the humanities, I felt like an intruder and soon began to compare the experience to learning a new language. It was humbling, to say the least. Soon, my head was spinning with words like gastrulation, embryogenesis, gamete, ectoderm, trophoblast, neural tube, mesoderm, just to name a few of those terms that I still remember. At the same time that this terminology was foreign to me, however, it was embedded in a narrative structure that was deeply familiar as it resembled many of the stories that I, as a professor of literature, taught regularly. Cells were presented as the protagonists in a story that took many twists and turns alongside the way to a fully formed human at the end of a nine-month period. Cells were "motivated," I soon learned, and they "migrated" along an arduous path, crossing "bridges," "aqueducts," "canals," "junctions," "ridges," and "crests." And, during their journey, they visited "domes" and even traveled across "polar" arteries. The cell's adventures in many ways resembled those of Homer's Odysseus, whose peripatetic travels figured prominently in the survey of European literature course that I was teaching at the same time. The language that we as humans use to describe the world, including biological processes, is that of human action. Anthropomorphization therefore serves as a powerful, if problematic, tool for understanding the nonhuman or, in the case of the cell, the small particle that constitutes a human.

As the semester progressed, I eagerly awaited the lecture on the development of the urogenital system. Reading eighteenth-century medical case histories on so-called “hermaphrodites,” I was intent on dispelling the mythical explanations that eighteenth-century scientists, despite all assertions to the contrary, often still upheld. Surely, nowadays, scientists understood what was *really* going on, I said to myself, looking, somewhat condescendingly, at the misinterpretations of our predecessors. Soon, however, phrases such as “appear to,” “should be,” and “not fully understood” emanated from the lectern. Even today, there are many gaps and ambiguities in science’s understanding of the different steps that transform an undifferentiated cell mass to a fully formed human. My initial expectation to get unambiguous answers clearly was misguided. It was unsettling to realize that, when entering the medical lecture hall, I had initially bracketed my usual critical stance toward disciplinary discourse, just because it was not my own. The history of science and medicine might appear as a teleological narrative with the present as the epistemological pinnacle, yet a closer look reveals that present-day science is riddled with as many uncertainties, contradictions, and mistakes as its prior incarnations. Like Odysseus, scientists often roam the vast ocean of information only to land in the same place of uncertainty from which they originally set sail.

My own journey into the realm of eighteenth-century “hermaphrodites” would be more arduous than I had expected. There was no undisputed truth to be culled from present-day medical discourse with which I could simply and unequivocally contrast the mistakes of the past. At the same time, uncovering the past became more important in order to understand present-day constructions of individuals whose bodies are deemed nonstandard in medical and popular discourse. This understanding has implications not only for these particular individuals but for all realms in which our embodied experiences matter, such as reproductive rights, gender-neutral bathrooms, racial bias, and informed consent, just to name a few of those topics that currently permeate popular and political discussions.

Medicalizing Difference presents the outcome of a journey that would not have been possible without the support and generosity of many. My institution, the University of Illinois, has provided generous research support during the research and writing of this book. My colleagues from my departments and from the Medical Humanities research cluster provided the necessary intellectual stimulation and a sounding board for this project at its various stages. Thank you to my friends who, during the isolating time of the early pandemic, bundled up to go on walks with me or to sit outside in sometimes frigid weather. Thank you to the editorial team at Bloomsbury and to the outside readers for their support of and constructive feedback on this project at its various stages. Most of all, thank you to my husband, who, as always, has been there every step of the way. And to my daughter who, during the time of writing this book, started out as a clump of undifferentiated cells who were motivated enough to migrate across many ridges, bridges, and crests on their journey to become the wonderfully rambunctious and funny human being that she is.

Introduction

Overview

In 1761, in the French town of Grenoble, Anne Grandjean successfully petitioned the court to become Jean-Baptiste Grandjean. Citing an error in the sex determination at birth, Grandjean was legally declared a man and married Françoise Lambert. In 1764, however, a former lover accused Grandjean of being a so-called "hermaphrodite." As a result, Grandjean was sentenced to the pillory, forced to wear women's clothes, and prohibited from having any contact with Lambert.

In eighteenth-century Europe, medical practitioners used the term "hermaphrodite" to designate a person whom they considered to have nonstandard sexual anatomy and variable sex characteristics, with a focus on the external genitals. The origin of the term lies in Greek mythology. The word "hermaphrodite" invokes the Greek myth of Hermaphroditus, Hermes and Aphrodite's son, who became two-sexed after the nymph Salmacis fell in love with him and fused her form with his. Even though eighteenth-century medical discourse, as part of Enlightenment science, explicitly distanced itself from mythological explanations of the natural world, it used and appropriated this term.[1] The word "hermaphrodite" circulated widely both in legal and popular writings. What exactly constituted a "hermaphrodite," however, was a subject of intense debate in which many of the prominent physicians of the eighteenth century participated. Rather than merely describing and analyzing a fact, these debates created their object of study.

The eighteenth century is a crucial time period between earlier conceptions of "hermaphroditism" and present-day notions of intersexuality (a term that I explain below). Retracing the history of the term is important not only to understand the construction of bodies as "hermaphroditic" but also to denaturalize related concepts of masculinity and femininity. In *The Shape of Sex* (2021), Leah DeVun surveys conceptions of nonbinary sex and their intersections with the notion of "hermaphroditism" from late Antiquity to the early modern period. Early Christianity embraced the idea of nonbinary sex through the idea of an androgynous Adam: "Beginning in late antiquity, certain Christian theologians described Adam as sexually undifferentiated, a lost prototype of human nature that reflected divine innocence and simplicity at the beginning of time" (17). Sexual un-differentiation was seen as the "original and most pristine state of humanity" (17). Over time, this concept merged with the image of the "hermaphrodite" from Greek mythology. Both terms were, for example, used synonymously by Augustine.[2] Over the course of the Middle Ages, however, the term "hermaphrodite" acquired negative connotations and those referenced were considered to "provok[e] the judgment of God" (28). In the early modern period, the connotations changed yet again when "alchemical literature used an image of a 'hermaphrodite' to describe a chemical agent believed to transmute base metals into gold and silver" (164). This notion converged with the concept of the "Jesus hermaphrodite" (164) and signified a "re-embrace of nonbinary sex parallel to that of early Christianity" (164).[3]

This brief historical survey of the period preceding the eighteenth century demonstrates the shifting signifieds associated with the signifier "hermaphrodite" and the multiple intersections with other conceptions of nonbinary sex. Both the term "hermaphrodite" and its referent are historically contingent constructions. "Hermaphrodites" were not simply "there"; rather, they were constructed in specific forms in different contexts. Their construction was intertwined with the predominant goalposts for masculinity and femininity in a particular historical and cultural setting. As Annemarie Mol has argued in her influential book *The Body Multiple* (2003), "Objects come into being—and disappear—with the practices in which they are manipulated" (5). The body itself means different things at different times; its constituent parts include not only anatomical structures but also, depending on the context, elements invisible to the naked eye such as hormones, chromosomes, and genes that are made legible through historically and culturally specific analytical practices. *Medicalizing Difference* builds on Mol's "move … away from epistemology … [which] asks whether representations of reality are accurate" (vii) and reflects on "medicine's *ontological politics*: a politics that has to do with the way in which problems are framed, bodies are shaped, and lives are pushed and pulled into one shape or another" (viii; emphasis in original). "Hermaphroditic" bodies, which were literally shaped by the medical establishment, highlight the ontological politics of a particular time period. These ontological politics gave rise to, in Ellen Samuels's words, "fantasies of identification," which seek

> to definitely identify bodies, to place them in categories delineated by race, gender, or ability status, and then to validate that placement through a verifiable, biological mark of identity. Fantasies of identification share certain signifying features: they claim a scientific, often medical framework and function to consolidate the authority of medicine yet in practice often exceed or contradict any actual scientific basis … And because they are fantasies, they merge imagination and the real through desire, a desire that manifests in material effects on actual people's bodies and lives. (2–3)

The particular eighteenth-century fantasies regarding bodies with nonstandard sexual anatomies—often equated with an individual's external genitals—led to their classification as "hermaphrodites" in medical discourse. These "fantasies of identification" were embedded in a discourse that consciously fashioned itself as purely scientific, yet it was constituted by the imagination and desire of those who produced it.

Current Debates

Following the lead of Hilary Malatino's research on "intersex ontology," *Medicalizing Difference* proposes to trace "hermaphrodite ontology" in the eighteenth century, the period often considered to be the precursor to present-day conceptions of the body. It explores the representation of "queer corporealities: bodies that don't cohere according to cis-centric, sexually dimorphic, ableist conceptions of somatic normalcy" (2). As Iain Morland, one of the contributors to the May 2022 "Intersex Issue" of *Transgender Studies Quarterly* argues, "Sexual difference is a structure or spacing between bodies rather than a bodily attribute" (166). Therefore, sexual difference "cannot be viewed from any given perspective, since each perspective belongs to a subject" (165) but is only discernible from the impersonal position of the gaze. Morland, writing from a Lacanian vantage point, posits that this impersonal position is occupied by "the subject position of surgery, [which] despite being only a single point, allows genitals to be seen as though from the nonplace of the gaze" (166). Developments in the realm of medicine, and in particular changes in the professional status of surgery, discussed in Chapter 1, make the eighteenth century a crucial time period for understanding the perception and construction of nonbinary bodies, in particular those perceived as "hermaphrodites." In this sense, *Medicalizing Difference* is a contribution to

> critical intersex studies, which has cohered only recently as a discrete academic specialization, [and] has points of overlap with the realms of medical ethics and medical humanities, gender studies, and science

> and technology studies, and has been shaped by two fundamental, often interwoven, foci: the construction of medical histories of intersexuality and the generation of activist interventions in the field of contemporary intersex diagnosis and treatment. (Malatino 3)

Medicalizing Difference closely reads case histories from the second half of the eighteenth century, a time period when the volume of writings on "hermaphrodites" increased considerably; the first case history discussed in this book was published in 1741 and the last one appeared in 1802. It thereby seeks to contribute to the understanding of not only the history of nonbinary bodies but also the medical discourse within which their representation was embedded. This reading practice ultimately allows for the critique of current practices of surgically normalizing those bodies that are seen as not fitting binary conceptions of corporeality.

It is important to reiterate that "what such intersex diagnoses share is not a common genetic, bio-chemical, or physiological etiology. Rather, intersex diagnoses share a failure to classify the body as male or female" (Wolff et al. 143). Intersex has therefore become, as David Rubin posits, "an umbrella term for the myriad characteristics of people born with sexual anatomies that various societies deem to be non-standard" (1). As one of the pioneering scholars of intersex, Morgan Holmes, posits, "Intersex, contrary to the dominant medical story currently in play, is a historical phenomenon and not a neutral biological fact. Intersex, as a set of bodily possibilities, has been both an object and product of knowledge for scientists and researchers who have made careers out of first identifying and then 'fixing' the 'problem'" (*Intersex* 31). Highlighting the historicity of the way in which bodies are perceived and shaped is front and center of critical intersex studies, which adopts a "reflective and reflexive mode" (Holmes, *Critical Intersex* 1) to highlight that intersex is "not one but many sites of contested being, temporally sutured to biomedical, political and social imperatives at play in each moment" (2).

While there are many convergences between intersexuality and eighteenth-century concepts of "hermaphroditism," they do not overlap seamlessly. A significant amount of scholarship has been published on intersexuality in the twentieth and twenty-first centuries, from a medical, legal, or cultural perspective. Much of it was triggered by activists writing against the practice of surgically "correcting" genitals that were deemed nonstandard, which began in the 1960s and 1970s and continues to the present day.[4] Anne Fausto-Sterling's *Sexing the Body* (2000), a pioneering study of gender politics and the construction of sexuality, traces the prevalent medical opinion that nonstandard genitalia in a newborn constitute a "medical emergency" (275–6) and therefore need to be altered surgically in childhood. As a reaction to this pathologization in medical discourse and practice, the Intersex Society of North American (ISNA) was founded in 1993. ISNA activists such as Cheryl Chase cautioned parents and medical practitioners against performing normalizing surgeries during childhood by emphasizing the notion of informed consent. In 2008, the ISNA was replaced by the Accord Alliance, which substituted the term "intersexuality" with "disorders in sex development," a terminology that has since then been questioned because it characterizes sexual ambiguity as a "disorder."[5] Cultural critics and medical activists such as Chase, Milton Diamond, David Griffiths, Peter Hegarty, Morgan Holmes, Katrina Karkazis, Suzanne Kessler, Hilary Malatino, Iain Morland, Erik Parens, Sharon Preves, Susan Stryker, Sharon Systma, and Bruce Wilson and W. G. Reiner have been deeply involved in the current ethical debates regarding the medical "management" of intersex people.

As a result of the shifting signifieds attached to the signifier intersex, critical intersex studies are inextricably bound up with transgender, queer, and feminist studies. Talia Mae Bettcher points out that, in the 1990s, "early transgender and intersex theory/politics were inevitably facilitated by the queer theory and politics of the day … Intersex theory/politics, while queer-inflected, arose in very close relation to the newly emerging trans theory/

politics" (410). Delving deeply into these debates in an attempt to demarcate the boundaries between these different concepts is beyond the scope of this project. Rather, *Medicalizing Difference* acknowledges their intersectional nature, also for the study of nonbinary bodies in the eighteenth century. As Jack Halberstam argues, "Trans* and intersex studies ... have the power to destabilize normalization, rendering the elusive 'normal' the only true 'abnormal'" (in DeVun and Tortorici 671).[6]

While the framework of intersex/queer/transgender/feminist studies is productive for the analysis of eighteenth-century conceptions of "hermaphrodites," one needs to heed Halberstam's caution against a "coloniality of the present" when looking at the past: "So rather than taking knowledge from our current context and using it as a template for the past, we must recognize how much we do not know about gender variability now and use that as a tool for withholding the imposition of knowledge onto vastly different cases from the past" (677). The goal of *Medicalizing Difference* is therefore an ontological one; through an investigation of the eighteenth-century pathologization of nonbinary sex, it invites the reader to critically examine present-day debates not only about intersexuality but also about embodied experience in general. In this respect, *Medicalizing Difference* acknowledges the fact that "what it means and has meant to have a legible body in the West—at least since the early modern period—has relied, in ways both straightforward and subtle, on the utilization of intersex bodies as impossible objects, as limit-figures that become interred in the ground upon which legitimate, recognizable, and acceptable sexed bodies are built" (Malatino 4). The eighteenth-century medical construction of "hermaphrodites" as limit-figures has much to teach us about sex and gender not only in medical discourse of the past but also in the present. My use of the now obsolete term "hermaphrodite" neither endorses nor normalizes eighteenth-century constructions of these bodies as deviant. Following Anne Linton's lead in *Unmaking Sex*, I use quotation marks around the term "hermaphrodite," which has "been perceived as traumatic and/or offensive to many contemporary intersex people" (4), to indicate that I am referring to eighteenth-century usage and to disrupt its implications.[7] Through the practice of reading medical texts against the grain—against their authors' overt intentions—*Medicalizing Difference* seeks to recover the embodied experience of those whose bodies were labeled as "hermaphrodites" beyond the medical description of the violent physical examinations to which they were subjected.[8]

The "Encyclopedic Age"

The late seventeenth and eighteenth centuries saw a gradual rejection of the early modern period's re-embrace of nonbinary sex. Whereas in the late medieval and early modern periods, individuals who did not fit the predominant norms of femininity and masculinity typically decided on their identity themselves, in the eighteenth century, physicians began to play an increasingly important role, leading to a gradual erasure of the "hermaphrodite's" agency.[9] Intent on establishing a purely secular basis for their inquiries, Enlightenment thinkers distanced themselves from interpretive frameworks that drew on Christianity and Greek mythology. They did, however, keep using the term "hermaphrodite." The "hermaphrodite" entry in the *Encyclopédie*, the Enlightenment reference work par excellence, is telling in this respect. Its author, Louis de Jaucourt, asks the central question regarding the possibility of human "hermaphrodites": "But are there true *hermaphrodites*?" ["Mais y a-t-il de véritables *hermaphrodites*?"] (165; emphasis in original). The first part of his answer is that, unlike in the animal and plant world, there are no "true" human "hermaphrodites" who can be either male or female in the reproductive process—such as most snails—because "there is nobody in whom the two sexes are perfect" ["il n'y a personne en qui les deux sexes soient parfaits"] (165).[10] The second part of Jaucourt's answer refers back to Greek mythology and states that there is no real-life Hermaphroditus. Nature may sometimes play hide-and-seek with the investigator, but "enlightened people" ["[des] gens éclairés"] (165) "in enlightened centuries" ["dans des siècles éclairés"] (165) who possess "true genius" ["véritable génie"] (166) can see through nature's "extremely strange games" ["jeux fort étranges"] (166) and uncover whether the so-called "hermaphrodite" is, in fact, either man or woman. In this entry, Jaucourt constructs the Enlightenment natural philosopher as capable of solving any riddle. At the same time that these comments crystallize the time period's programmatic belief in science, they also thinly veil an unacknowledged awareness of, to use Ellen Samuels's phrase, the "fantasies of identification" that shape its inquiries.

During the eighteenth century, which I have elsewhere called the "Encyclopedic Age," all forms of ambiguity, ambivalence, and liminality were supposed to be classified away and thereby erased.[11] The desire to "unmask" "hermaphrodites" as either male or female mirrored the consolidation of the sex/gender binary during this time period. This dichotomy was mapped onto a concurrent solidification of the binary regarding the public and the private sphere. The sphere of the "public" was equated with "masculine" and "political," whereas the realm of the "private" was associated with "feminine" and "domestic."[12] These overlapping binaries index the anxieties of a time that was undergoing momentous social and political upheaval, culminating in the French Revolution and its pan-European ramifications in the form of the French Revolutionary Wars.[13] Any blurring of the boundaries between masculine and feminine and public and private was perceived as threatening, as can be seen in the eighteenth-century reactions to other nonbinary figures such as cross-dressers, effeminate male characters, and female husbands.[14] In her analysis of the "female husband" in eighteenth-century discourse, for example, Jen Manion highlights the multiple intersections between different types of trans positions in the eighteenth century, including "hermaphroditism," which "challenged essentialist understandings of sexual difference" (1). As Julia

Ftacek argues, recovering "transness" in the eighteenth century "calls on us to investigate the underpinnings of biological essentialism" (311) and to lay bare the simultaneous codification and bending of gender norms in eighteenth-century writing, whether literary or medical. Eighteenth-century medicine's construction of nonbinary bodies as "hermaphrodites" needs to be carefully historicized in order to expose the underlying "fantasies of identification." This historicization is particularly productive if deployed side by side with current theories regarding gender/sex, race, class, and ability that open up eighteenth-century medical texts to be read against the grain.

Twentieth-and twenty-first-century studies of gender and sexuality have triggered interest in earlier, in particular nineteenth-century, "hermaphrodites." Michel Foucault's 1978 edition of the memoir written by Herculine Barbin (1838–68), along with the accompanying medical documents, was particularly influential in this respect. In Foucault's edition, published as *Herculine Barbin dite Alexina B.*, Foucault combined a sociohistorical approach with textual analysis to trace the representation of Barbin as a "hermaphrodite" in nineteenth-century medical and popular discourse. One of the most influential critics to emerge in this analytical tradition was Alice Dreger, whose pioneering study *Hermaphrodites and the Medical Invention of Sex* (1998) posits that the nineteenth century was the Age of Gonads. In this time period, scientists dissected gonadal tissue during autopsies with the goal of identifying either ovarian or testicular markers under the magnifying lens of the microscope. Dreger provocatively posits that, in the nineteenth century, because "non-emergency exploratory surgeries were quite rare, and biopsies basically unheard of ... the only true hermaphrodite was a dead hermaphrodite" (Dreger, *Intersex* 9). Only the "hermaphrodite's" death gave the nineteenth-century scientist the promise of certainty. Geertje Mak's *Doubting Sex* (2012) follows a similar investigative path by locating the origins of twentieth- and twenty-first-century normalizing surgeries in nineteenth-century microscopic examinations of gonadal tissue. In their analyses, both Dreger and Mak highlight that these laboratory exams provided much less clarity than expected and therefore muddled the scientists' conclusions. Building on their work, Anne Linton's *Unmaking Sex* (2022) explores this ambiguity by examining the interdependence of literature and medicine in the nineteenth century, arguing that "literary representations of 'hermaphroditism' are … in fact, awash with the same cultural and historical anxieties as medical case studies" (3).

While there exists a significant amount of scholarship on "hermaphroditism" and intersexuality from the nineteenth century to the present day, much less attention has been paid to the eighteenth century and its role in shaping contemporary attitudes toward individuals whose sexual anatomy medical and popular discourse considers nonstandard. While the earlier part of the eighteenth century is often subsumed in discussions of the early modern period, the latter part tends to be constructed as a precursor to the nineteenth century. Studying the eighteenth century and its treatment of "hermaphrodites" in its own right is, however, crucial because of the particular conditions that shaped the production and dissemination of knowledge, which continue to influence research and treatment practices to the present day. As Londa Schiebinger argues, the eighteenth century

> saw the emergence of modern science, (what we have come to call) scientific sexism related to modern notions of femininity and masculinity, and scientific racism. This triad—science, and scientific notions of sexual and racial differences—emerged not as disassociated and unencumbered phenomena, but as developments that formed each other in decisive ways. (*Nature's Body* xi)

The eighteenth century therefore marks a pivotal moment in the medical construction of "hermaphrodites," which was embedded in evolving notions of gender and race, as well as developments in the scientific and political realm.

Establishing hierarchies and classifications—the Linnean system being the most prominent one—was a sign of the Enlightenment's search for scientific answers to centuries-old questions about the natural world. This development had a significant impact on the study of individuals with nonstandard sexual anatomy. In this context, scholarship typically presents the eighteenth century as a turning point in moving these bodies from the mythological to the scientific and medical realms.[15] This argument largely follows Michel Foucault's in *Les anormaux* (1974–5), which emerges from his observations regarding the classical episteme in *Les mots et les choses* (1966). Foucault posits that, during the eighteenth century, the necessity of a scientific discourse on sexuality emerged. According to Foucault, because this discourse was heteronormative, case histories on "hermaphrodites" denied sexual ambivalence by classifying bodies with nonstandard sexual anatomies as either male or female, typically according to their sexual orientation. While it is true that the authors of most eighteenth-century case histories on "hermaphrodites" purport to have uncovered the "true" sex of the individual they study, their doubts surface repeatedly and thereby undermine any statements of certainty. They seek to codify the sex and gender binary yet at the same time bend it, which is a process largely ignored by Foucault. In *Les anormaux*, Foucault appears to take the eighteenth-century impetus for classification at face value, contradicting his own conclusions regarding the ambiguities found in eighteenth-century medical examinations of individual patients in *Naissance de la clinique* (1963): "Classificatory thought gives itself an essential space, which it proceeds to efface at each moment. Disease exists only in that space, since that space constitutes it as nature; and yet it always appears rather out of phase in relation to that space, because it is manifested in a real patient, beneath the observing eye of a forearmed doctor" (*Birth of the Clinic* 9). Discussing the Grandjean case mentioned at the beginning of this introduction, Foucault posits that eighteenth-century taxonomies classified "hermaphroditism" out of existence. However, a closer look reveals that even though eighteenth-century medical men—and they were all men—claimed certainty, their texts are marked by doubt and unanswered questions. The more closely scientists looked at living "hermaphrodites," the more complex their classificatory project became. This complexity triggered the writing of yet more case histories, which in turn further undermined any attempt at scientific definitiveness. The publication of these case histories thereby paralleled the development of Linnaeus's system of classification, *Systema Naturae*, which swelled from the originally planned 12 to 1,300 pages (LaFleur 2) or that of the *Encyclopédie*, which, a mere four years after the publication of its final installment, necessitated a *Supplément* (Hilger, "Orientation" 173). Each case history gave rise to another one that revised the conclusions of its predecessors, thereby revealing the ambivalences of the Enlightenment project.[16]

Current Scholarship

The ramifications of Foucault's argument and its limitations can be seen in Thomas Laqueur's *Making Sex: Body and Gender from the Greeks to Freud* (1990), one of the most influential monographs discussing gender and sexuality. *Making Sex* posits that an important shift occurred over the course of the eighteenth century, namely, the transition from the one- to the two-sex model of gender. The one-sex model, which had dominated scientific thinking since the writings of the Roman physician Galen in the second century, posited the sexes on a continuum. Women were considered inferior versions of the male ideal and were thought to possess the same biological structures as men, only in an inverted or incomplete version. The vagina was, for example, seen as an inverted penis. Over the course of the eighteenth century, however, this homology was questioned and woman was constructed as man's complete opposite.[17] In this context, the vagina was no longer understood in analogy to the penis; it instead became a mysterious organ that the Enlightenment scientist needed to scrutinize.[18] Rather than serving as an argument for equality, however, the difference between men and women was interpreted hierarchically and served to consolidate the gender binary and, consequently, the domestication of women in the private sphere.

For the analysis of eighteenth-century "hermaphrodites" in particular, Laqueur provides a seemingly neat explanatory framework, not least because his thesis aligns with both Foucault's argument in *Les anormaux* and the Enlightenment's classifying and hierarchizing mission itself. As the two-sex model gradually replaced the one-sex model and the gender binary consolidated, each supposed "hermaphrodite" was classified as either male or female. There was no longer any space for individuals who did not fit the prevailing norms for masculinity and femininity. Laqueur, however, downplays many of the tensions in eighteenth-century thinking about gender and sexuality in general and nonbinary individuals in particular. His thesis has been critiqued by historians and cultural critics such as Leah DeVun, Katharine Park and Robert Nye, and Michael Stolberg, among others, who argue that these changes did not occur abruptly over the course of the eighteenth century and that the one-sex model endured and itself contained contradictions. The focus on elite scientific and medical texts is another criticism wielded at Laqueur's argument. Because eighteenth-century case histories on "hermaphrodites" typically address a double audience, medical professionals and a popular readership interested in natural history, they provide particularly fertile ground for nuancing Laqueur's thesis. The analysis of these case histories highlights the intersections between the one- and the two-sex model and the contradictions within the Enlightenment project of establishing clearly demarcated classifications.

Even though important strides have been made in the study of other nonbinary individuals in the eighteenth century, there exists comparatively less research on those who were called "hermaphrodites" during this time period. In this respect, *Medicalizing Difference* is indebted in particular to the work by Ruth Gilbert (2002), Patrick Graille (2001), and Maximilian Schochow (2009), who survey and discuss eighteenth-century fictional, medical, and legal writings in the British, French, and German context, respectively. Albeit from different vantage points, all three authors highlight the increasing importance of medical discourse in creating the category of the "hermaphrodite" in the transnational scientific networks of the eighteenth century. *Medicalizing Difference* builds on their work by discussing the case history, the genre of choice for medical experts.

The Case History as a Genre

As Gianna Pomata has shown, medical case histories have existed in some form or other since the time of Hippocrates. During the early modern period, they developed into *observationes* and *curationes* and became fully institutionalized in the context of the eighteenth-century professionalization of medicine.[19] As Enlightenment scientists (a term that I will use to refer to all areas of inquiry that we nowadays describe as science)[20] and physicians focused on empirical knowledge, case histories began to play an increasingly important role in the collection, creation, and dissemination of knowledge. They used the genre to posit the empiricism of their observations and professional identity in contradistinction to the imaginative, mythological accounts of their predecessors, thereby striving to establish a clear demarcation between science/medicine on the one side and literature on the other. These scientists and physicians wrote in a genre that sought to set itself apart from belles lettres through its empirical focus. However, their writings demonstrate that the line between these case histories and imaginative writing was much more permeable than they themselves realized or were willing to acknowledge.

At the same time that case histories are associated with eighteenth-century science and medicine, they also share characteristics of other emerging eighteenth-century genres. In this context, Nicolas Pethes ascribes the development of the German *Bildungsroman* to the same interest in the empirical aspects of an individual's development and a "redefinition of literature as referring to reality" (29): "Literary case histories appear as novels (such as *Werther*), intradiegetic parts of novels (such as the harpist in *Wilhelm Meisters Lehrjahre*), whole-life biographies (*Anton Reiser*), fragmentary details of a crisis (*Lenz*), dramatic scenes (*Woyzeck*), or magazine articles (Poe, Warren)" (41). The presence of case histories in literary texts demonstrates the pervasiveness and impact of this genre in cultural consciousness. In his study of the medical case history and the British novel, Jason Tougaw posits that the "case history is medicine's answer to the Enlightenment call for empiricism, and the novel is literature's answer. Writers in both genres experimented with techniques that could give narrative shape to identity, and over the course of two centuries, the genres influenced each other by exchanging both subject matter and methods" (2). As Tougaw demonstrates in his readings of nineteenth-century British fiction, the case history and fiction borrow from one another in complex and interdependent ways:

> While the novel relies on the conventions of realism to signify its fictionality, the case history relies on the conventions of fiction to create the illusion of total mimesis. But the representation of living, breathing human beings becomes a burden to the writers of case histories, calling attention to two troubling realities: that illness is intrinsic to life and often eludes the power of medical science. In response, medical writers consistently turn to novelistic conventions that provide aesthetic resolutions in the absence of scientific ones. By the same token, novels borrow the mantle of empiricism. (15)

The empirical interest in an individual, often in unusual or extreme circumstances, unites case history and the novel, both of which want to tell "a good story." Tougaw's observations are certainly applicable to the eighteenth century, which programmatically established itself as an empirical age. With respect to case histories about "hermaphrodites" in particular, these convergences between the genres are all the more important because, in contrast to nineteenth-century medical publications on "hermaphrodites," which mainly reported dissections of gonadal tissue from deceased individuals, eighteenth-century case histories were predicated on a living and breathing "hermaphrodite." Writing about a living individual necessarily imbued eighteenth-century case histories with an element of open-endedness. The fact that a particular physician's case history often did not end in scientific resolution led to the production of "sequels," follow-up studies by different physicians, that, like serialized fiction of the time, kept the interest of a growing reading public alive with the promise of more revelations and salacious details. These texts were marketed to a growing readership and circulated widely. Audiences were as eager to learn of a "hermaphrodite's" fate as they were to read about the trials and tribulations of fictional characters in eighteenth-century novels.

Eighteenth-century case histories on "hermaphrodites" blur the line between science and belles lettres at the same time that they seek to consolidate it.[21] In this respect, eighteenth-century case histories offer "an alternative to disciplinary antagonism" (Class ix) and their history is "a viable alternative to disciplinary contradistinction, offering ample room for genuine encounter and even giving us glimpses of past indivisibility" (vii)[22] Taking the argument about the case history's hybridity one step further also allows for a questioning of present-day disciplinary specialization and the separation of knowledge into the sciences and the humanities, which is typically seen as a fact rather than a historical construct, mainly of the nineteenth century. In particular, this vantage point allows for a reconsideration of medicine in this dyad. Rather than being a hard science, medicine is an interpretive practice, similar to many humanities disciplines, in which the human body figures as a text that needs to be read and interpreted. These interpretations give rise to what Catherine Belling has called, "hermeneutic anxiety" (376) that informs not only medicine's practice but also all of its textual productions, from the past to the present day.

Critical Intersex Studies and Medical Humanities

In this respect, *Medicalizing Difference* offers a contribution not only to critical intersex studies but also to calls for questioning the divide between literature and medicine, in particular, and the sciences and the humanities, more broadly.[23] The most forceful calls for bridging these disciplinary separations already occurred in the 1970s as a reaction to the transformation of medical schools into high-powered research centers in the previous decade. These calls resulted in fields such "literature and medicine," "narrative medicine," "medical humanities," and "health humanities," which have become institutionalized through professional organizations, publications, curricula, professorships, and academic centers over the course of the past three decades. However, much of the scholarly work in these fields centers on the twentieth and twenty-first centuries.[24] From this perspective, the divide between the sciences and the humanities appears as an immutable reality. Approaching the effort to connect the sciences and the humanities from an eighteenth-century vantage point, however, demonstrates that the separation of these realms of knowledge, and its institutionalization, is a relatively recent phenomenon. The eighteenth century constitutes a transitional period between the de facto interdisciplinarity that had reigned until the early modern period and the separation of the sciences and the humanities that was institutionalized in the European system of higher education in the nineteenth century and its eventual global dissemination by way of Anglo-American research universities in the twentieth century. Eighteenth-century thinkers reacted to the beginnings of this disciplinary specialization, when the Cartesian mind-body dichotomy was mapped onto the separation of the humanities and sciences, which were eventually characterized as "soft" and "hard," respectively.

Eighteenth-century case histories on "hermaphrodites" illustrate the tension between the onset of disciplinary specialization and the continuing interdisciplinarity which presented a more holistic approach to human experience and, by implication, the human body. Authors strove to position themselves firmly on the side of science by highlighting their empiricism, yet by doing so, they also unwittingly invoked conventions from imaginative narrative genres from which they want to distance themselves. Whereas most scholarship has read eighteenth-century medical case histories from a scientific or historical perspective in an essentially descriptive way, uncovering these tensions requires a reading of these texts that goes against the grain of their authors' intentions. As Tod Chambers argues in the *Fiction of Bioethics*, case histories need to be read as complex narratives. Authors might state that a certain "hermaphrodite" is a man or a woman, yet a close reading of their narratives, which are themselves positioned on the permeable boundary between fictional and scientific writing, uncovers the underlying ambivalences, doubts, and contradictions.[25] In an era that was undergoing tumultuous social, political, and cultural change, inquiries into "hermaphrodites" posed questions regarding not only sex and gender but also race and ability. Close textual readings, coupled with insights from embodiment studies, show that at the same time that these case histories sought to consolidate binaries they questioned them.

Intersectional Embodiment Studies

Reading eighteenth-century case histories about "hermaphrodites" against the grain therefore not only mobilizes intersex studies and the contiguous fields of feminist, gender, queer, and trans* studies, it also intersects with other areas of embodiment studies, in particular disability and critical race studies. In *Disability Theory*, Tobin Siebers explores the intersectional and overlapping nature of identities:[26] "The theory of complex embodiment views the economy between social representations and the body not as unidirectional as in the social model, or nonexistent as in the medical model, but as reciprocal" (25). "Hermaphrodite" bodies are the terrain on which different identities intersect; they thereby demonstrate that embodiment is not only reciprocal but also multidirectional. Jack Halberstam, for instance, mentions disability studies in addition to trans* and intersex studies as one of those approaches that "have the power to destabilize normalization" (in DeVun and Tortorici 671). In *Narrative Prosthesis*, David Mitchell and Sharon Snyder argue that disability has the "unambiguous ability to impact every other identity category at the same time" (x). In this sense, disabled bodies are what Rosemarie Garland-Thomson calls "extraordinary bodies": "Constructed as the embodiment of corporeal insufficiency and deviance, the physically disabled body becomes a repository for social anxieties about such troubling concerns as vulnerability, control, and identity … Disability, then, is the attribution of corporeal deviance—not so much a property of bodies as a product of cultural rules about what bodies should be or do" (6). The fact that "both the female and the disabled body are cast as deviant and inferior" (Garland-Thomson 19), along with the defective male body (Wiehe), has important implications for the construction of "hermaphroditism" in the eighteenth century, situated as it was on the border between normative femininity and masculinity and between ability and disability. Jason Farr's study of disability and sexuality in eighteenth-century British literature "expose[s] able-bodiedness and heterosexuality as imbricated systems that sustain dominant models of reproductive futurity" (1) and concludes that "impaired bodies are thus fundamental to the cultural construction of homo- and heterosexuality" (2). Questions regarding the "hermaphrodite" body's reproductive potential—its potential disability—are front and center in eighteenth-century medical case histories. Sex/gender and (dis)ability need to be thought together, along with race and class, in order to understand the intersectional and multidirectional ways in which identities were constructed during the Enlightenment.

In *The Limits of the Human* (2003), Felicity Nussbaum explores the "cross-hatched representations of race, gender, and anomaly" (1) in imperial England.[27]

She observes a "defective and racialized femininity that paradoxically energizes an imperial England as it struggles to demarcate the limits of the human through women" (2). In the eighteenth century, individuals whose sexual anatomies were considered nonstandard were often described as monstrous women. This monstrousness was projected onto those remote lands that European nations were in the process of colonizing and whose inhabitants were typically described as less human than their European counterparts. This discourse, which intersected with the Enlightenment project to classify the natural world, provided the ideological justification for the economic basis of slavery by aligning it with emerging notions of racial difference. At the same time that alterity was projected onto foreign lands, racial difference was also displayed and spectacularized at home, on the stage, and in other public places. Enslaved bodies were stared at and consumed, not unlike exotic objects in eighteenth-century consumer culture, such as coffee, tea, and cocoa (Kowaleski-Wallace). Ramesh Mallipeddi shows how these moments of "spectacular suffering" establish "the problem of slavery as a problem of embodiment" (3). The presence in European cities of the bodies of African slaves, whose presumed lack of reproductive capacity projected them into the realm of disability, generated a similar type of anxiety as the ingestion of foreign consumer goods. Both blurred the lines between femininity and masculinity, ability and disability, and European versus non-European.[28] As the work of the above quoted scholars demonstrates, the field of postcolonial studies has much to contribute to this discussion as scholars "have yet to come to grips with the relation between the Enlightenment and the creation of a global world" (Outram 8).[29]

Questions of Agency

Medicalizing Difference examines mid- to late-eighteenth-century medical case histories on "hermaphrodites" from three different languages and contexts—British, French, and German. Scientists and physicians publishing in these languages and circulating in the territories in which these languages were spoken were part of what Gianna Pomata has called a "network of exchange" ("Sharing Cases" 197) in which ideas and publications circulated extensively. Tracing these debates in this particular network broadens the discussion beyond the predominant Anglophone focus.[30] This, in turn, highlights the fact that writings on "hermaphrodites" were shaped by specific contexts and that medical men communicated their research in strategic ways across national and linguistic boundaries. A comparative approach to the construction of the "hermaphrodite" therefore shines a spotlight on how authors from different contexts imagined a "normal" body and, thereby, a "healthy" citizenry.

In order to be able to perform close readings against the grain, *Medicalizing Difference* focuses on those case histories written about four specific individuals: an unnamed Angolan "hermaphrodite," Maria Dorothea Derrier, Michel Anne Drouart, and Anne Grandjean, published in the time period 1741–1801. The amount of eighteenth-century writings *about* these "hermaphrodites" stands in stark contrast to the absence of writings *by* them. This lack was noticed already during the eighteenth century, when the poet Édouard-Thomas Simon (1740–1818), who was also a physician, felt compelled to publish a fictional letter by Anne Grandjean—discussed in Chapter 2—in an attempt to give a voice to the person who was the topic of intense debate in the medical and popular press.

The absence of writings by "hermaphrodites" forces us to consider one of those intersectional identities rarely explored in scholarly discussions, namely that of class. European "hermaphrodites" who became objects of eighteenth-century medical discourse all hailed from the lower classes of society. Some of them had to consult medical specialists when their physique was perceived as nonstandard by their surroundings. Others exhibited their bodies to provide financially for themselves or their families after other avenues for securing an income had failed. Enslaved "hermaphrodites" from non-European territories were displayed for a fee by their owners. While there are significant differences between these individuals, they were all most likely illiterate. There is therefore no eighteenth-century equivalent to Herculine Barbin, whose writings can be read side by side with the medical case histories about them. In this context, Jason Farr reminds us that "class also determines one's experience of physical disability and intellectual achievement" (135). Unlike the famous author Alexander Pope who, disabled by Pott's disease, could assert his agency through his writings, Grandjean, Drouart, Derrier, and the unnamed Angolan "hermaphrodite" were not in a position to actively resist and respond to medical professionals.[31] In contrast to their counterparts from the laboring classes and the peasantry, bourgeois and aristocratic parents were able to protect their children from the prodding and probing fingers of the medical establishment. In fact, at several points in their writings, medical men lament the fact that "hermaphrodites" from well-to-do parents were hidden from their inquisitive gaze.

The lack of direct "hermaphroditic" subjectivity in the eighteenth century is one of the aspects that makes the scholarly exploration of this topic an uncomfortable endeavor; it poses the question of the ethics of writing about those who have no voice. As Leah DeVun has observed in the context of researching medieval and early modern notions of nonbinary sex, "Activists and allies have been rightly critical of scholarship that uses people with intersex variations or transgender people *instrumentally*—that is, as mere bodies to 'think with'—and that, in the process, displays little consideration for people's actual perspectives and lived experiences" (*The Shape of Sex* 205; emphasis in original). Since "the voices of these past figures are all but lost to us" (205), the scholar discussing "hermaphrodites" from the Middle Ages to the eighteenth century experiences the same impasse as the postcolonial critic who wrestles with the absence of "colonized subjects whose writing might offer a history of anti-hegemonic and anti-colonial writing" (Kaul 424). The desire to find subaltern voices—to borrow a term from postcolonial scholarship—is particularly pronounced in discussions of "hermaphrodites" living during the period traditionally called the Enlightenment. Situated in-between the Middle Ages and the early modern period, on the one hand, and Herculine Barbin's nineteenth-century memoir and intersex activism in the twentieth and twenty-first centuries, on the other, the eighteenth century is a paradoxical time period. At the same time that the Enlightenment championed the human rights of liberty and equality, it also erased the agency of those who did not fit into a literalized notion of fraternity as a group of privileged men.

Reading against the Grain

In order to understand the Enlightenment's ontological politics regarding "hermaphrodites," medical case histories about them need to be read closely and against the grain, interrogating seemingly factual statements, questioning underlying assumptions, and exploring conspicuous silences. The close engagement with these texts forces us to engage their graphic descriptions of invasive physical exams and acknowledge their disturbing nature. As Eli Clare posits in his study of notions of normalcy and cure, *Brilliant Imperfections*, "Some of the fragments in this book are razor sharp. The histories, ideas, realities I'm grappling with are full of pain and violence, grief and rage" (xix). While this type of trigger warning, which was developed by feminists in the 1980s and 1990s, is necessarily incomplete since it is impossible to know everyone's trigger, it is a necessary first step toward disrupting the voyeuristic dimension of these texts. This disruption, in turn, paves the way for a discussion regarding the ethics of eighteenth-century physicians' construction of the "hermaphrodite" as an object of study. The goal of these close readings is not to concur with their diagnoses but, on the contrary, to counteract the re-medicalization of these bodies by demonstrating that the pen of the Enlightenment physician was as violent as the dissecting knife of the nineteenth-century scientist and the scalpel of the twentieth-century surgeon. In fact, as James McGuire points out, the Indo-European root of the Latin *scribere* (writing) means cutting and making an incision (111). The Enlightenment pen is the first in a series of steps oriented toward the medical "normalization" of bodies that were deemed nonstandard, which culminated in the 1960s and 1970s practice of surgically reshaping them. Unpacking the ways in which eighteenth-century medical men wielded their pen to put their intrusive and violent examinations onto paper reveals that these liminal bodies are "extraordinary" in the two senses discussed by Garland-Thomson. At the same time that they become a "repository for social anxieties" (6), their "superabundance" (xi) makes it difficult to contain them within the pages of a single case history, necessitating the production of further writings. It is precisely in "hermaphroditic" bodies' destabilization of the categories established by the Enlightenment pen that glimpses of their subjectivity emerge. "Hermaphrodites'" bodies function in a similar way as "tropicopolitans," which is a term used by Srinivas Aravamudan to describe figures of anticolonial resistance. Eighteenth-century "hermaphrodites" and imperial subjects are both liminal figures who, because of their subaltern status, have no direct voice with which they can respond to those who construct them as other. Their agency can only be found through a complex task of close reading that centers on those moments when they question and disrupt the pathologizing discourse of those who attempt to control them.

In a work on "hermaphrodites," the use of pronouns poses a linguistic challenge. We only have texts *about* "hermaphrodites" and not *by* them, making it all but impossible to access their embodied experience directly. Additionally, in their texts about "hermaphrodites," physicians were not always consistent in their use of pronouns. Their conclusions regarding their subject's sex did not always match the pronoun that they used, which is significant in itself as it signals their ignorance of the embodied experience of the individuals whom they studied. Also, since *Medicalizing Difference* discusses texts written in French and German, it is important to note that some of the gendered linguistic features of pronouns and adjective endings get lost in English translation. In French, in contrast to English and German, possessive pronouns take the gender of the noun they modify, making it unclear at times whether an author is referring to an individual as male or female. These linguistic ambiguities undermine eighteenth-century medical men's biological essentialism, despite their forceful and repeated assertions to the contrary. In an acknowledgement of the blurring of binary concepts of sex and gender by those whom the medical establishment labeled as "hermaphrodites," *Medicalizing Difference* will employ the gender-neutral and gender-inclusive pronoun "they." This pronoun was not in use during the eighteenth century and "hermaphrodites" were forcefully assigned as either male or female. However, using "they" in a twenty-first-century work of scholarship acknowledges the fact that we do not know how these individuals conceived of their identity at the same time that it attempts to recover their agency as extraordinary individuals who, in Garland-Thomson's sense, questioned the boundaries that were imposed upon them.

The Cases

The core corpus of *Medicalizing Difference* consists of the medical case histories, written in English, French, and German by multiple authors, about Maria Dorothea Derrier, Michel Anne Drouart, Anne Grandjean, and an unnamed Angolan "hermaphrodite." These four "hermaphrodites" will be discussed throughout the four chapters, which will put the various studies about them—a total of nineteen—into dialogue both within and across chapters. The writings on these four individuals are indicative of the ways in which the eighteenth-century medical establishment constructed "hermaphrodites" as their object of study. The following pages serve as a guide to their stories, yet readers are urged to remember that the "facts" themselves are shaped by the ontological politics regarding sex and gender in the eighteenth century.

The *Angolan* "hermaphrodite" remains nameless in the oldest text discussed in this book, James Parsons's *A Mechanical and Critical Enquiry into the Nature of Hermaphrodites* (1741). The individual in question was transported on a slave ship from their home in Angola to North America and from there to Bristol before being put on display in London. Except for the fact that they were twenty-six years old at the time of their arrival in the British capital, nothing is known about their life. In his treatise, Parsons uses the exhibit as a platform to explore earlier claims that "hermaphroditism" can be found with greater frequency in hot climates by aligning it with aberrant female sexuality. Even though Parsons strives to locate "hermaphrodites" firmly in foreign lands, the movements of the Angolan "hermaphrodite" in the Atlantic world project them into the British realm and thereby set the stage for subsequent case histories on European "hermaphrodites."

Assigned female at their birth in Grenoble, France, in 1732 *Anne Grandjean* legally became Jean-Baptiste at the age of fourteen due to their genitalia. After living as a man for a number of years in precarious financial circumstances, Grandjean was accused of being a "hermaphrodite" by a former female lover. Grandjean was sentenced by the court of Lyon and subsequently imprisoned. Grandjean appealed the judgment in Paris and was incarcerated there. In 1765, the lawyer Vermeil wrote a "mémoire" in defense of Grandjean's decision to live as a man. In response to this document, the lawyer Champeaux argued that Grandjean was a biological woman and should therefore live as one. Grandjean's appeal was only partly successful. On the one hand, they were found not guilty of having profaned the marriage sacrament and were therefore released from prison. Yet, on the other, Grandjean was ordered to wear women's clothes, their marriage was annulled, and they were prohibited from having any contact with their former wife.

In contrast to Grandjean who was assigned female at birth, *Michel-Anne Drouart*'s first name, which combines male and female components, established the newborn as a "hermaphrodite." Like Grandjean, Drouart, born in 1733 or

1734, was raised as a girl. Later in life, however, Drouart consulted authorities at the Sorbonne, who recommended a legal sex change to male, yet doubts regarding their physique persisted. The Drouarts's home was visited by curious contemporaries as news of their child's "hermaphroditism" spread. Drouart's parents, stocking weavers with several other children to support, eventually sent their child to a surgeon in London who exhibited Drouart for a fee. This led to a lifetime of Drouart traveling throughout Europe, displaying their body to various medical professionals.

In 1801, *Maria Dorothea Derrier*, the 22-year-old daughter of poor laborers, visited the Charité hospital in Berlin in search of treatment for a case of scabies. In the process of giving their patient a therapeutic bath, physicians deemed Derrier's genitals to be nonstandard. This assessment set off a vigorous debate, in which some of the most renowned medical men of the time participated. Like Drouart, Derrier traveled throughout Europe before eventually settling in Bonn as a man, alternatively called Karl Derrier or Charles (Carl) Dörge.

Medical men such as Christoph Wilhelm Hufeland, Sauveur François Morand, and James Parsons entered into dialogue with each other, discussing these four individuals in nineteen case histories; they did so within and across historical periods and national boundaries. Their case histories form a dense textual web that sheds light on discussions about sexuality and gender that are embedded in a number of interrelated shifts in the way knowledge was generated and disseminated in the eighteenth century: the professionalization of medicine in conjunction with the increasing demand for empirically produced knowledge, the expanding market for popular scientific literature, changing notions about generation and reproduction, and the exploration of foreign territories. Each of the four chapters in *Medicalizing Difference* builds on the previous one and explores the effect of one of these shifts on the ontological construction of the "hermaphrodite" in the context of eighteenth-century discourses on race, gender, class, and ability.

For ease of reference, the two tables in the appendix provide (1) in alphabetical order by author, the list of publications on the four "hermaphrodites" discussed in this book, including their authors' conclusion as to the supposed "true" sex of the individual whom they studied, and (2) the list of "hermaphrodites," with authors' conclusions regarding their sex. Reading medical men's writings about so-called "hermaphrodites" against the grain, highlighting the contradictions and ambivalences in their conclusions, allows us to disrupt the medical construction of this category and recover, in the absence of any writings by the "hermaphrodites" themselves, glimpses of their embodied experience.

Chapter Outline

Chapter 1, "Medical Empiricism," positions case histories on "hermaphrodites" in the context of the increasing demand for empirical research. The chapter begins with James Parsons's *Mechanical and Critical Enquiry into the Nature of Hermaphrodites* (1741) before proceeding to a close reading of the later case histories about Grandjean, Drouart, and Derrier, paying particular attention to the national and regional contexts in which these histories were published. Until the seventeenth and early eighteenth centuries, scientific literature mainly consisted of lengthy summaries and commentaries on previously produced writings, going back to Antiquity, typically without any firsthand scientific investigation. Prior to the eighteenth century, a stark distinction between university-trained physicians, who mainly possessed theoretical anatomical learning, and surgeons, who had acquired practical knowledge through apprenticeships, shaped all medical writing. Because of their association with barbers, surgeons tended to be less respected than physicians. With the increasing expectation that science be empirical, the modes of knowledge production changed and surgeons' professional reputation improved. Anatomical knowledge garnered from living bodies and corpses became valued currency in the medical field, leading to the creation of teaching hospitals with surgeon-physicians. The case history, with its detailed focus on one individual, became the privileged genre for both surgeons and traditional physicians to establish themselves professionally. With their case histories on "hermaphrodites," these practitioners competed with each other, seeking to establish and consolidate their professional standing in the medical realm. The construction of the "hermaphrodite" as an object of medical study is therefore intricately intertwined with medical men's self-fashioning in the eighteenth century.

Chapter 2, "Entertainment Science," discusses the exploding market for popular science in the eighteenth century. Case histories on "hermaphrodites" became a financially and professionally profitable venture as they allowed authors to tap into a market where books on natural history, written in the vernacular rather than Latin, became bestsellers. At the same time that the authors of case histories strove to establish their writings as scientific in contradistinction to more popular types of literature, such as the novel, they drew on some of the same narrative conventions employed in those genres. Focusing on the case histories about Drouart, in particular those by Burghart, Delius, and Vacherie, this chapter explores the empirical voyeurism and erotic empiricism that emerges as a result of the power imbalance between physician and his object of study.

Chapter 3, "Reproduction: Fluids and Other Matters," situates eighteenth-century research on "hermaphrodites" in broader debates about generation and reproduction, in particular the theories of preformation and epigenesis, by focusing on the case histories on Drouart by Hoin, Morand and Ferrein: In their quest to assign "hermaphrodites" their "true" sex, scientists devoted much time trying to determine their reproductive potential. Their inquiries were embedded in broader national debates about the role of men and women in generating a healthy citizenry. In addition to the visible external genitals, they investigated bodily emissions such as semen and menstrual fluid. However, the ambivalent meanings of these fluids, which were often still considered in the context of humoral medicine, thwarted scientists' attempts to find conclusive answers. The description of "male menstruation" in particular undermined any efforts at establishing a clear binary, as did physicians' oftentimes intrusive and painful physical exams, which highlighted the power differential in these medical encounters.

Chapter 4, "Terra Incognita/Parts Unknown," posits that the anxiety caused by liminal bodies, including "hermaphrodites," was displaced onto tropical climates, which were seen as being particularly conducive to blurring the line between masculinity and femininity. Those same territories were the object of imperial fantasies in the eighteenth century. The wish to understand "hermaphrodites" and erase their ambiguity dovetails with the desire to conquer foreign territories and the bodies inhabiting them, a process that was represented in highly gendered, racist, and ableist language. The reading of Parsons's text, in particular his dissection of a female fetus, and of Monorchis's case history on Derrier shows how the imperial commodification of consumer goods was extended to those deemed to display aberrant femininity and who were consequently described as "hermaphrodites." This context highlights the fact that writings on "hermaphrodites" not only address issues of sex and gender but also engage with emerging theories on race.

Appendix

Table 1 List of Publications by Author, with Their Conclusions Regarding the "Hermaphrodites'" Sex

Burghart, D. Gottfried Heinrich	*Gründliche Nachricht an seinen Freund ****	1763	Drouart	F(emale)
Champeaux, Claude	*Réflexions sur les Hermaphrodites*	1765	Grandjean	F

Delius, Heinrich Friederich	"Nachricht von dem besondern Hermaphroditen Drouart."	1765	Drouart	M(ale)
Des Essarts, Nicolas-Toussaint	*Procès fameux*	1788	Grandjean	M
Ferrein, Antoine	*Mémoire sur le véritable sexe*	1767	Drouart	F
Hoin, Jean Jacques	*Nouvelle Description*	1761	Drouart	F
Hufeland, Christoph	"Beschreibung und Abbildung"	1801	Derrier	F
Martens, Franz Heinrich	*Beschreibung und Abbildung*	1802	Derrier	M
Mayer	"Description Anatomique d'un Hermaphrodite connu"	1836	Derrier	Undecided
Mayer	"Description of An Hermaphrodite"	1836	Derrier	Undecided
Mertrud, Antoine	*Hermaphrodite, Dissertation*	1749		
Monorchis, F. F.	"Von dem neuangekommenen Hermaphroditen"	1801	Angolan Drouart Derrier	F F F
Morand, Sauveur-François	"Description d'un hermaphrodite"	1750	Drouart	M
Mursinna, Christian Ludwig	"Von einer besondern Naturbegebenheit."	1801	Derrier	F
Parsons, James	*A Mechanical and Critical Enquiry*	1741	Angolan	F
Simon, Edouard-Thomas	*L'hermaphrodite*	1765	Grandjean	M
Stark, Johann Christian	"Kurze Beschreibung"	1801	Derrier	M
Vacherie, M.	*An Account of the Famous Hermaphrodite*	1750	Drouart	Undecided
Vermeil, F. M.	*Mémoire pour Anne Grandjean*	1765	Grandjean	M

Table 2 List of "Hermaphrodites," with Authors' Conclusions Regarding Their Sex

Angolan "hermaphrodite"
Monorchis: F(emale)
Parsons: F
Derrier
Hufeland: F
Martens: M(ale)
Monorchis: F
Mursinna: F
Stark: M
Drouart
Burghart: F
Delius: M
Ferrein: F
Hoin: F
Monorchis: F
Morand: M
Vacherie: Undecided
Grandjean
Champeaux: F
Des Essarts: M
Simon: M
Vermeil: M

Notes

1 "Hermaphrodites" were no longer understood in the context of mythology but were "taxonomized as a natural anatomical anomaly" (Epstein, "Either/Or" 117), which "powered the move of gender disorders from the realm of the monstrous into the natural realm" (116).

2 Jacqueline Murray similarly explores nonbinary sex in her work on monasticism as a third gender in the Middle Ages, as do the contributors to Alicia Spencer-Hall and Blake Gutt's collection, *Trans and Genderqueer Subjects in Medieval Hagiography* (2021).

3 For a discussion of the perception of "hermaphroditic" bodies in the Middle Ages and the early modern period, see, for example, Ruth Gilbert, Kathleen Perry Long, Jenny Mann, Christof Rolker, and François Soyer.

4 In this context, Morgan Holmes spells out the medical establishment's literal phallocentrism:

> It is a peculiarity of postwar Euro-American medical discourse and practice that any child born with a clitoris measuring as small as .5 cm according to some reports ... and .9 cm in others ... but who has otherwise typically female internal reproductive organs—a complete cervix and vagina and unfused labia—can be diagnosed as a hermaphrodite and submitted for clitoral reduction surgery. (*Intersex* 36)

5 The term "intersex" replaced the word "hermaphrodite" in the late twentieth century, first in activist and then in popular and medical discourse. The Intersex Society of North America (ISNA), which was formed in 1993, defines intersex as a "variety of conditions in which a person is born with a reproductive or sexual anatomy that doesn't seem to fit the typical definitions of female or male" (Intersex Society of North America). The Accord Alliance, which was created in 2008, defines the concept of "disorders of sex development" (DSD) more broadly as "when a less common path of sex development is taken" (Accord Alliance, "Disorders of Sex Development"). As a possible reaction to criticism regarding the choice of the pathologizing term "disorder," the Accord Alliance's homepage also refers to DSD as "differences in sex development," which allows for keeping the same acronym while changing the terminology's implications (Accord Alliance, Homepage). Also see Holmes (*Critical Intersex*) on the debate in the shift in terminology from "intersex" to "DSD."

6 For a discussion of the tensions between trans* and intersex studies and communities, see the May 2022 issue of *Transgender Studies Quarterly*, in particular the introduction by Michelle Wolff, David Rubin, and Amanda Lock Swarr. Also see Iain Morland's essay in this journal issue on the possible collaboration between intersex and trans* studies to interrogate medicalization. With respect to the issue of medicalization, also see stef shuster's *Trans Medicine*.

7 My use of the terms "variable sex characteristics," "nonbinary sex," and "nonstandard sexual anatomy" to refer to eighteenth-century physicians' criteria for determining "hermaphrodites" is based on the current scholarship cited above and reflects the term's shifting signifieds. These terms always need to be thought within implicit quotation marks as what is considered "variable," "nonbinary," and "nonstandard" is historically and culturally contingent.

8 Scientists and physicians writing in English, French, and German all used the term "hermaphrodite." In French, "hermaphrodite" has a double grammatical gender ("le" or "la"), in an acknowledgment of its referent. The German "Hermaphrodit" has a male grammatical gender ("der") and was the predominant term used in the eighteenth century. By the mid-eighteenth century, "Hermaphrodit" had pushed the word "Zwitter," from the Old High German "zwitarn" ("consisting of two") to the sidelines in scientific discourse.

9 The agency of "hermaphrodites" in the late medieval period in particular is discussed in Rolker. Also see DeVun, "The Jesus Hermaphrodite" and *The Shape of Sex* on this issue.

10 It is important to note here that the term "hermaphrodite" to designate two-sexed animals is itself based on the Greek myth about Hermaphroditus.

11 See Hilger, "Orientation."

12 Jürgen Habermas's *Strukturwandel der Öffentlichkeit* (1962), translated as *The Structural Transformation of the Public Sphere* in 1989, famously theorized the construction of this binary in the eighteenth century. Since then, Habermas's theory has been critiqued and nuanced in its application. Habermas was criticized for projecting the British situation onto France and the German-speaking lands, which were different in their social and political structures. For the German context, see Peter Uwe Hohendahl, Isabel Hull, and Ernst Manheim. For France, see Dena Goodman and Rémy Saisselin. In addition, scholars objected to Habermas's construction of a bourgeois master narrative (Richard Sennett), his focus on the public sphere to the detriment of the private realm (Philippe Ariès and Georges Duby), his oversight of the role of gender in the public sphere (Elizabeth Eger et al, Joan Landes, and Johanna Meehan), and his neglect of such issues as race, nationalism, religion, science, and class (Guy-Uriel Charles and Luis Fuentes-Rohwer; Craig Calhoun). Also see Lincoln Dahlberg, Nancy Fraser, Andreas Gestrich, Michael Hofmann, and Simon Susen for syntheses of the critiques of Habermas's concept of the public sphere and his idealization of the liberal public sphere.

13 On this topic, see Hilger, *Gender and Genre*.

14 See Ula Lukszo Klein for an analysis of the "female cross-dresser as a third category of gender representation that challenges our understanding of gender and its relationships to desire and the body" (3). In *Gender and Genre*, I have similarly described the literary representation of the cross-dressed soldier during the French Revolutionary Wars in particular. Also focusing on a politically charged time period, Declan Kavanagh retraces the scandal involving member of parliament John Wilkes in

1750s and 1760s Britain and explores "how effeminacy figures as a discourse of crisis" (xvii).

15 In the discussion of the emergence of the modern self, Dror Wahrman, for example, argues that "hermaphrodites" "were mostly dismissed as fictions or turned into metaphors" (44) in the eighteenth century.

16 For a discussion of this process in the *Encyclopédie*, the eighteenth-century reference work par excellence, see Hilger, "Orientation."

17 The one- and the two-sex model represent the Hippocratic and the Aristotelian tradition, respectively. With respect to sexual difference, the Hippocratic tradition posited a continuum, whereas Aristotelian thinking established a system of binary oppositions. On this point, see Daston and Park, "The Hermaphrodite."

18 In *The Mind Has No Sex?*, Londa Schiebinger pursues a similar line of reasoning when she observes that this difference was thought to permeate not only genital anatomy but all aspects of the female body, including skeletal structures.

19 On this point, also see Class and Epstein, "Either/Or" and "Historiography."

20 The word "scientist" was only coined in the first half of the nineteenth century. In the eighteenth century, those who performed scientific research writ large were referred to by a variety of terms such as natural philosophers, *encyclopédistes*, naturalists, and so on. For ease of reference, in my (meta)discussion of the eighteenth century, I will use the present-day term "scientist" for all those performing research relating to humans and their environment. "Scientist" is therefore always to be read with implicit quotation marks.

21 See Hilger, "Introduction."

22 For innovative scholarship investigating the interpenetration of the literary sphere and the scientific realm, see the publications by Courtney Smith, Helen Thompson, and Tita Chico (all). For work on medical case histories in particular, the work by Sandra Pott, Rudolf Behrens and Carsten Zelle, and Susanne Düwell and Nicolas Pethes is particularly helpful.

23 In reference to C. P. Snow's influential *The Two Cultures and the Scientific Revolution* (1959), the separation between the sciences and the humanities is often described as the two-culture debate.

24 For a more extensive discussion of interdisciplinarity in the eighteenth century, see Hilger, "Medical Humanities."

25 In this respect, *Medicalizing Difference* extends the conclusions made by Courtney Thompson regarding the visual elements, which are an integral part of case histories on "hermaphrodites," to the textual components: "scholarly certainties in this period about the existence or nonexistence of the hermaphrodite were often belied by visual depictions of hermaphrodites, which were caught between practices of scientific, artistic, and pornographic illustration" (392–3).

26 Siebers takes Patricia Hill Collins's observation regarding the "tendency of identities to construct one another reciprocally" (Collins 212, in Siebers 27) as a starting point to explore the multiple identities with which disability intersects.

27 In this respect, also see Deutsch and Nussbaum's edited collection, "*Defects.*"

28 See Sussman for a discussion of these anxieties in the context of the emerging British opposition to slavery.

29 The fraught relationship between postcolonial theory and eighteenth-century colonialism is the topic of Daniel Carey and Lynn Festa's edited collection, *The Postcolonial Enlightenment* (2009).

30 For another such network, the Spanish-Portuguese one, see De Souza, Soyer, and Vicente.

31 See Helen Deutsch for a discussion of Alexander Pope's writings in the context of his disability.

1

Medical Empiricism

Men-Midwives

The ontology of the "hermaphrodite" as a category in eighteenth-century discourse is closely intertwined with developments in the medical realm. Over the course of the eighteenth century, firsthand, empirical ways of knowing were increasingly valued and began to replace earlier ways of knowledge production, which mainly consisted of lengthy summaries and commentaries on previously produced writings, going back to Antiquity. In the eighteenth century, physical examinations of deceased and living individuals became increasingly common and constituted the basis for case histories, which presented and circulated this knowledge. These case histories were seen as presenting pure facts, while older treatises were considered as nonfactual, fictional, and even mythological. Surgeons, because of their direct encounter with the human body, began to play an increasingly important role in the medical realm, which they entered most forcefully through, what in present-day terms would be called, the field of obstetrics and gynecology. In this context, the genre of the case history, which is embedded in the self-fashioning of surgeons as premiere medical experts, plays an important role in the construction of the "hermaphrodite" as an object of medical study.

The Scottish caricaturist's, Isaac Cruikshank's, frontispiece[1] to Samuel Fores's *Man-Midwifery Dissected; or, the Obstetric Family Instructor*[2] (1793) crystallizes these developments. Cruikshank depicts the man-midwife as an uncanny creature, split into two parts: on the left, a male with gynecological instruments and pharmaceutical remedies in a vaguely institutionalized medical setting and, on the right, a woman standing in front of the hearth in a private home.[3] Cruikshank's drawing illustrates the eighteenth-century public's ambivalence about the presence of a male in the birthing chamber, a space traditionally reserved for women. Male practitioners were typically only called in cases of emergency, when the use of the forceps or other surgical tools became necessary.[4] Over the course of the eighteenth century, however, these men increasingly sought to assert their presence, even during uncomplicated births.[5] Their first patients were women from the lower classes, often in a hospital setting.[6] Helping these women imbued physicians with a sense of altruism. In the context of "Enlightenment humanitarianism" (Lindemann, "The Discourses" 397), "Charitable work … became a standard ethical accoutrement for an enlightened physician who aspired to honor, distinction, and affluence" (395). Gradually, however, men-midwives assisted in the births of bourgeois and aristocratic women, for whom the presence of a male physician in their home not only brought the promise of medical expertise but also signified social and financial status. As Adrian Wilson has shown, surgeons strove to transform medicine, in particular obstetrics, into a male-dominated profession through the exclusion of female health practitioners. At the same time that these men gradually strengthened their position as obstetricians, critical voices cautioned pregnant women, and their husbands, against excessive surgical intervention. The fact that Laurence Sterne's eponymous hero Tristram Shandy describes the damage done to his nose by Dr. Slop's forceps is indicative of the general unease with these types of intervention. In addition, critics of man-midwifery cautioned women about the inappropriateness of a male in the birthing chamber. In Cruikshank's caricature, contemporaries' fear of the morally corrupt doctor is represented by the love potions standing on a shelf amidst a vast array of pharmaceutical remedies.

The incursion of male physicians into the birthing chamber was a gradual and slow process. Therefore, in practice, most childbirths in the eighteenth century still occurred in the presence of female midwives, whose ability and credentials were judged by the female community through a complex process of consensus building.[7] Consequently, midwives were typically the ones who decided on the sex of newborns with external genitals that were deemed nonstandard. As the eighteenth century progressed, however, medical men began to assert themselves as authorities in these cases. These men tended to be surgeons with obstetrical expertise, whose skill set either intersected with or was equivalent to that of the emerging man-midwife.[8] This development further contributed to the professional devaluing of midwives, whose testimony regarding bodies with variable sex characteristics gradually became inadmissible in court. Lisa Forman Cody argues that these surgeons "proclaimed an objective point of view that allowed them to transcend the intense and subjective experiences of pregnancy and childbirth" (294). This objectivity is, as Iain Morland has pointed out in his writings on intersex and the construction of sexual difference, claimed by "the subject position of surgery, [which] despite being only a single point, allows genitals to be seen as though from the nonplace of the gaze" (166). Surgery's self-presentation as an objective and disengaged discipline obscures the fact that the eighteenth-century medical gaze did not merely observe but actively constructed its objects of study.

Surgeons' professional reputation improved during the eighteenth century, yet their position remained precarious not only because of the continued presence of midwives in the birthing chamber but also because the status of surgery itself remained contested in the eighteenth century. With their case histories on those they constructed as "hermaphrodites," surgeons strove to position themselves in a gradually changing medical sphere. The resulting pathologization of bodies that eluded simple binary classifications with respect to gender, race, and ability is intertwined with surgeons' fears regarding their own tenuous professional identity. It is in this sense that Cruickshank's depiction of the man-midwife/surgeon as a half-male/half-female individual, a "hermaphrodite" of sorts, intersects with eighteenth-century medicine's construction of "hermaphrodites" as objects of study and bodies in need of medical intervention. Eighteenth-century surgeons' "fantasies of identification" regarding "hermaphrodites" "claim a scientific, often medical framework and function to consolidate the authority of medicine yet in practice often exceed or contradict any actual scientific basis … [as] they merge imagination and the real through desire" (Samuels 2–3). Surgery claims scientific objectivity yet is profoundly shaped by its practitioners' own subjectivities.[9] As a result, in their efforts to assert their own agency, surgeons erased the embodied experience of those whose physique they scrutinized.

Surgeons and Physicians: Experience and Theory

In the eighteenth century, two main groups were licensed to practice medicine, surgeons and physicians. The training and education of surgeons mainly occurred in the context of an apprenticeship. As Roy Porter observes, surgery was "judged a manual skill rather than a liberal science" (*Greatest Benefit* 277). By contrast, physicians were considered gentlemen. They were educated at a university and were part of a corporative system of professional associations, which granted medical licenses, typically for a specific geographical area. Whereas surgical training emphasized practical knowledge of the human body, academic medical education focused on reviewing and evaluating medical knowledge published since antiquity.[10] During the eighteenth century, however, the strict separation between surgeons and physicians gradually began to erode, leading to a "rapprochement between medicine and surgery" (Bonner 56). Surgeons strove to become respected members of the medical profession and therefore gradually separated from barbers, with whom they had been associated since the Middle Ages, and founded their own professional associations.[11] Part of surgeons' increasing professionalization consisted of attending courses at private medical schools and hospitals. Conversely, university-trained physicians, who mainly possessed theoretical anatomical knowledge, increasingly participated in anatomical dissections. Empirical anatomical knowledge of the human body became valuable currency in the medical field.

The gradual fusion of practical and theoretical knowledge of the human body occurred throughout Britain, France, and the German territories, yet there were significant national and even regional differences. Whereas in Britain and France, practical knowledge was gained outside the university, in Germany it was acquired within. French surgeons had a better reputation than their German counterparts and they eventually created their own professional corporations. Generally, in France and Germany, the state had a bigger role in the medical realm than in the Anglo-Saxon context, where private entrepreneurship was more pervasive in both the teaching and practice of medicine. Developments were rather uneven, both across and within different national contexts, especially in German lands, which lacked a unifying political center.[12] As a result, medicine remained unregulated by contemporary standards, as can be seen in the numerous practitioners who worked outside the medical hierarchy, ranging from quacks, charlatans, and mountebanks to unlicensed women physicians, so-called petticoat doctors. Publishing firsthand observations on controversial and salacious medical cases, such as "hermaphrodites," served as a way for a medical professional to establish his reputation and thereby increase the revenue potential of his practice in this evolving professional context.

The increasing emphasis on empirical knowledge of the human body shapes James Parsons's *Mechanical and Critical Enquiry into the Nature of Hermaphrodites*. Published in 1741, this text is situated at a crucial point of transition between traditional forms of knowledge production—commentaries on previous scholarship—and research in the form of direct examinations of human bodies. Parsons highlights the empirical impetus for his project in the preface, when he mentions a "female Fœtus that came to [his] Hands" (iv). He presents the fetus as the trigger for his inquiry into human "hermaphroditism," which is guided by the goal that "the Truth, which hitherto has been so clouded and obscured on this Head, may be said at least to begin to dawn" (ix). In line with his empirical focus, in his signature, Parsons identifies himself as a "Fellow of the Royal Society," which was founded in the seventeenth century with the goal of promoting empirical inquiry; he even dedicates his *Enquiry* to its president, Sir Hans Sloane. Parsons, who was educated in Paris and graduated from Rheims with a medical degree in 1736, continued his training in London under James Douglas, whom he describes as the "most consummate Anatomist" (133).[13] Assisting Douglas, who practiced as an obstetrician, in his anatomical studies allowed Parsons to gather significant firsthand knowledge of the human body, especially of the female reproductive system. Parsons's report on his dissection of a female fetus in *Enquiry* represents the intersection of his empirical interests with the field of obstetrics, which he himself would eventually practice.

With his case history on the fetus, Parsons distances himself from mythological explanations for "hermaphrodites." He thereby represents the "profound mutation in the self-definition of intellectuals. For them wonder and wonders became simply vulgar, the very antithesis of what it meant to be an homme de lumières, or for that matter a member of any elite" (Daston and Park, *Wonders* 18–19). Parsons couches his empirical project in a language replete with Enlightenment metaphors. The actual discussion of the fetus, however, does not occur until his concluding chapter and is, at a mere ten pages, comparatively short. In-between his preface and his conclusion stand 140 pages that do not constitute an empirical inquiry into human "hermaphroditism" but a review of and commentary on writings on the topic since antiquity, which was the traditional way of knowledge production up to the early modern period. Parsons argues that "it was quite necessary to examine what authors had said on that Head" (v) in order to debunk the "doctrines, founded by the Ancients upon the most absurd Principles" so as to achieve "the Expulsion of superstitious Mysteries and Errors, and, in fine, the Promotion of Truth" (iv). *Enquiry* thereby functions as an encyclopedic "reader's digest," quoting, paraphrasing, summarizing, translating, and popularizing previous treatises on the topic of human "hermaphroditism." Parsons's literature review acknowledges the fact that, by the mid-eighteenth century, the amount of publications on the topic of human "hermaphroditism" was copious and therefore needed to be synthesized. At the same time that this literature review grounded Parsons's argument, its length—which far exceeded that of his own empirical research—demonstrates that the shift to purely empirical modes of knowledge production was still incomplete in the mid-eighteenth century, despite the Royal Society's efforts.[14]

Parsons's dissection of the fetus represents surgeon-anatomists' gathering of knowledge through postmortem examinations. At the same time that medical professionals examined corpses, they also became increasingly interested in the workings of the living human body. The fact that Parsons juxtaposes the dissected fetus with the examination of the individual whom he calls "Angolan" and who will be the focus of the fourth chapter, is paradigmatic in this respect. The interest in the functioning of living bodies represents a shift from mechanistic to vitalistic modes of interpretation:[15]

> Mechanists … looked at the body in terms of a machine or mechanism, and were interested in finding out how all the parts fitted together and how they worked, much on the model of the notorious clock. Dissection and anatomy were crucial tools for this approach, and the *Encyclopédie* article on anatomy has a very strong mechanist heritage. Vitalists rejected this on the basis that the body was something more than a mechanism interpretable according to the combined laws of mechanics, hydraulics,

> chemistry and physics. They argued that it required a dedicated science of "life" to understand the body properly, and that it was only by observing life processes, that is to say, by not examining it once life was extinct, that anything could truly be discovered about it. (Warman 98)

Eighteenth-century surgeon-anatomists discussing "hermaphrodites" did not merely dissect corpses but also established themselves as authorities on living bodies. They did so through the genre of the case history and thereby asserted their expertise in the determination of individuals with nonstandard sexual anatomy, as can be witnessed in the 1765 court case of Anne/Jean-Baptiste Grandjean.

Assigned the female sex at birth in Grenoble, France, in 1732, Anne Grandjean legally became a man at the age of fourteen. A former lover's accusation that Grandjean was a "hermaphrodite" set in motion a legal process. Grandjean was sentenced to three days in a straightjacket with a sign around the neck that read "desecrator of the sacrament of marriage" ["profanateur du sacrament de marriage"] (Graille 132).[16] In addition, Grandjean was banished from their hometown of Lyon. Grandjean appealed the judgment in Paris and was transferred to a prison there. The well-respected lawyer François-Michel Vermeil wrote a defense of Grandjean's legal sex change and argued for Grandjean's right to continue life as a man. Vermeil's defense was questioned by another lawyer, Claude Champeaux, who posited that Grandjean was a biological woman and should continue to live as one. While neither lawyer was involved in the trial itself, which was widely followed beyond the medical and legal realm, their publications shaped public opinion, which, in turn, affected the outcome of the case.

Both lawyers invoked the expert opinion of surgeons, attesting to the profession's rising status. Vermeil references the "report by the physicians and surgeons from Lyon" ["Procès-verbal de visite des Médecins & Chirurgiens de Lyon"] (14), whom he does not name. He inserts the relevant part from the report, which was written in Latin but does not translate it, presumably "out of tactfulness" ["par délicatesse"] (14). Instead, he paraphrases it in a way that bolsters his defense of Grandjean's life as a man. Champeaux, in agreement with the condemnation of Grandjean by the court of Lyon, starts his study with a praise of the practice of surgery, underlining its empirical dimension: "Surgery, that central part of the healing arts, only believes what it has seen and examined; hermaphrodites need to be relegated to Ovid's metamorphoses" ["la Chirurgie, cette partie essentielle de l'art de guérir, n'a voulu croire que ce qu'elle a vu et examiné; les hermaphrodites doivent être relégués dans les metamorphoses d'Ovide"] (6). Champeaux pastes the same paragraph from the surgeon's report into his document as Vermeil. He, however, questions its authenticity (38)—associating it with the realm of mythology—by juxtaposing it to a different surgical report, signed by "Brac, Docteur en Médecine, Faissole & Champeaux" (43). The signature reveals that Champeaux, a lawyer with surgical expertise, was present at the exam, which concluded that the examiners found "nothing else that differentiates the so-called Grand-Jean from other women" ["rien autre qui distingue ladite Grand-Jean des autres femmes"] (43). Champeaux presents the Latin report included by Vermeil as invalid and even fraudulent; he performs a word-by-word—"mot à mot" (38)—refutation that argues that none of the key phrases in the excerpt are in the actual report from which they were supposedly taken. Both lawyers invoke empirical knowledge gathered by surgeons as an objective position from which to argue their case. Yet this objectivity is embedded not only in the surgeons' "fantasies of identification" but also in the lawyers' subjectivity and alignment with specific ideological positions, which led to the selective and strategic use of excerpts.

The Grandjean trial ended with the Paris court issuing a new sentence that established a compromise, which sought to reconcile the opposing viewpoints. Even though Grandjean's marriage was annulled, the court of Lyon's judgment that Grandjean profaned the sacrament of marriage was overturned. The mitigation of Grandjean's sentence can be attributed to the fact that, as Vermeil argues throughout his defense, Grandjean acted “de bonne foi” (21), in good faith, after having been legally reassigned as a man and that the surroundings had accepted the new identity. However, when Grandjean was released from prison, Grandjean was ordered to wear female clothing and forbidden from “haunting” [“hanter”] (23) their wife and other women (see Graille 129–44). The court’s use of the word “hanter” encapsulates the eighteenth-century anxiety about identities that unsettled neat classifications and were relegated to the realm of the uncanny, which needed to be observed and controlled.

Power

The role that law and medicine played in shaping the lives of those viewed as “hermaphrodites” points to the power differential that rendered the production and dissemination of medical case histories possible in the first place. Like Grandjean, whom Vermeil describes as being “born into poverty” [“né dans la pauvreté”] (Vermeil 20), and the first patients treated by men-midwives, “hermaphrodites” typically hailed from the lower social strata and experienced financial precariousness. This hardship made them subject to exploitation by surgeons, who medicalized their bodies as objects of study for their own professional benefit and thereby erased their subjectivity.[17]

The case of Michel-Anne Drouart illustrates the importance of social class particularly forcefully. Drouart, born in 1733–4 in Paris, was baptized Michel-Anne, a hyphenated name that contains masculine and feminine components, and was raised as a girl. Authorities at the Sorbonne, whom Drouart consulted later in life, legally reassigned Drouart as male. For an individual growing up in precarious circumstances, this reassignment created broader employment opportunities. Drouart became an apprentice to a toy-painter, but this career path proved “ineffectual, through the constant Interruptions and Visits which the Report of the child being an Hermaphrodite, drew upon it from all Quarters, insomuch as the parents, who, though not very easy in their Circumstances, had not the least Idea, at that Time of exposing it to View, for any Advantage or Lucre, thought themselves obliged to take it Home" (Vacherie 5). After taking their child home, Drouart's parents, stocking-frame weavers with several other children to support, allowed curious contemporaries to visit, as news of Michel-Anne's unusual genitalia spread. They eventually sent their child to a surgeon, identified as "Mr. Fage'aise" (Vacherie 6), who exhibited Drouart for a fee at his home. After being exhibited in France, Drouart was put on display in Carnaby Street, London, in November 1750. Drouart spent the remainder of their life traveling throughout Europe, displaying their body to various medical professionals, which resulted in multiple case histories. While none of the reports address the question of payment explicitly, Vacherie, a surgeon from Brussels who published his case history after visiting Drouart in London, hints at the financial necessity that propelled Drouart to become an object of study for medical men throughout Europe. Even though the issue of social status is never mentioned, it is the foundation for the construction of the "hermaphrodite" in the eighteenth century as witnessed by the fact that there are no aristocratic "hermaphrodites" to be found in the pages of these case histories. The rise of empirical medicine was inextricably linked to the existence of economically disadvantaged individuals. Medical examinations of these "hermaphrodites" catered to the voyeurism of medical professionals, for whom these case histories represented an opportunity to rise socially and economically, and to the voyeurism of the general public, who consumed these publications as entertainment.[18]

Textual Creations

Detailed physical exams became the basis for numerous publications on Drouart over a twenty-year period; each case history entered into dialogue with the documents produced previously, creating a dense textual web that captured the audience's curiosity in a similar way as the most popular serialized novels of the time. The main publications on Drouart are, in chronological order, those by M. Mertrud (1749), Sauveur François Morand (1749), M. Vacherie (1750), Gottfried Heinrich Burghart (1763), Heinrich Friederich Delius (1765), Antoine Ferrein (1767), and Jean Jacques Louis Hoin (1772).[19] In addition, Drouart's name can be found in numerous entries on "hermaphrodites" in reference works such as the *Encyclopédie* and the *Supplément à l'Encyclopédie*.[20] Drouart was a topic of discussion in the French, English, and German medical sphere and soon became a celebrity beyond the medical realm. While the various authors come to diametrically opposed conclusions regarding Drouart's sex, they all share the same anxiety about positioning themselves in the rapidly changing professional sphere of the eighteenth century. For them, Drouart becomes a vehicle to assert their credentials. Their professional agency is predicated on the erasure of their object of study's subjectivity.

Each author goes to great lengths to establish his credibility by emphasizing the empirical basis of his medical knowledge; they all underline their firsthand observation of Drouart's body. Morand prefaces his description by highlighting that "this is what I observed" ["voici ce que j'ai observé"] ("Description" 1). Delius similarly emphasizes that he reports only "what I myself observed" ["was ich selbst wahrgenommen habe"] (399) during an anatomical lecture in Nürnberg. And Vacherie underlines his active role when he mentions that he "sprea[d] the thighs" (10) and that his "exploring touch" (11) allowed him to "soun[d] deeper in" (11) than those before him, echoing the narrative conventions of eighteenth-century erotic literature, which will be explored at greater length in the next chapter. The case histories all share a similar format: they focus on the external genitals, which are measured, described in detail, and typically accompanied by an illustration. The empirical medical gaze selects and records; it brings the "hermaphroditic" body into being in a violently voyeuristic way that combines science and entertainment in a specifically eighteenth-century manner.

Vacherie, a surgeon from Brussels, examined Drouart in London and, in 1750, published his case history there, situating his text in the profitable English medical sphere.[21] In addition to the medical instruction available at universities, a veritable marketplace was emerging outside of the academic realm that satisfied the growing demand for empirical knowledge of the human body, in particular through anatomical demonstrations. In the wake of James Douglas's pioneering activities, anatomical demonstrators competed for customers, extensively advertising their offerings to a broad audience. Vacherie positions his study in this context, inviting the reader to join him in his empirical quest with a title page that resembles popular broadsides and promises an "Account of the Famous Hermaphrodite, or Parisian Boy-Girl, Aged Sixteen."

In addition to establishing the empirical basis for their observations, medical men typically foregrounded their membership in, and therefore recognition by, national professional associations and regional academies. In fact, their publications often appeared after their lectures at those societies' meetings (McClive 218). As Parsons's identification of himself as a fellow of the Royal Society shows, the emphasis on these affiliations and recognitions strove to bolster medical men's respectability and professional standing. In the signature of his text on Drouart, Mertrud, for example, describes himself as the "full-time royal surgeon, sworn in at St Côme by the Academy and anatomical and surgical demonstrator at the king's garden [the royal natural history museum]" ["chirurgien ordinaire du roi, juré à St Côme, de son Académie, et démonstrateur en anatomie et chirurgie au jardin du roi"] (n.p.), strategically referencing both his empirical knowledge gathering and his position at court. Similarly, Morand acted as the demonstrator of surgery, also at the *Jardin du Roi* in Paris.[22] Famous for the removal of kidney stones, Morand was one of Paris' premiere surgeons. He used the language of the Enlightenment to increase the social and professional standing of surgery. In 1743, he published a *Discours dans lequel on prouve qu'il est nécessaire au chirurgien d'être lettré* [Treatise in which it is proven that a surgeon needs to be lettered]. In this treatise, Morand argued that, in their training, surgeons should not focus exclusively on surgical techniques because those were skills that, according to him, could be acquired quickly. By contrast, he posited that they needed general medical knowledge as well as knowledge of classical languages, logic, and physics. In short, they needed to become lettered gentlemen, who, like their physician competitors, were educated in the liberal arts. With this treatise, Morand participated in the pamphlet warfare between physicians and surgeons in 1730s and 1740s Paris, from which the surgeons emerged victorious with two royal decrees. Consequently, French surgeons had raised their social status significantly by the mid-eighteenth century. As a specialist of the urogenital system, Morand's decision to participate in the scientific debate about Drouart served a strategic function. Published in 1749, at the end of the pamphlet warfare, his case history allowed Morand not only to strengthen his position in the crown-supported medical sphere but also to establish a foothold in the emerging medical marketplace.[23]

Knowledge Networks

Medical men were able to examine Drouart because Drouart traveled extensively not only in France but also throughout Europe. The transnational debate about "hermaphrodites" only became possible because their bodies appeared in front of medical men's inquiring gaze, typically driven by financial necessity. Gottfried Heinrich Burghart, the first German-language author to publish on Drouart, outlines Drouart's extensive travels:

> From the great number of passports and other papers that he carried, I gathered that his name was Michael Anna Drouet [*sic*] and that he was born in Paris. He had just arrived from Bartenstein in Prussia via Warsaw,

> from where he got the most recent passport, graved in copper, from the French envoy to the royal court there. He explained to me, half in French and half in German, which he knew somewhat, that he traveled throughout the world to exhibit himself to curious people as a wonder of nature.
>
> [Aus seinen in Menge bei sich habenden Paessen, und anderen Pappieren bemerckte ich, daß er Michael Anna Drouet [*sic*] hieße, und von Paris gebürtig sei. Jetzo kam er von Bartenstein aus Preußen über Warschau, von woher sein jüngster in Kupfer gestochener Paß, von dem am dasigen Königlichen Hofe stehenden französischen Gesandten lautete. Er gab mir halb französisch und halb Deutsch, mit welcher Sprache er sich etwas behelfen konnte, zu verstehen, daß Er in der Welt herum reisete, um sich als besondres Wunder der Natur, curieusen Personen zu zeigen.] (16)

The documents carried by Drouart testify to their complex travels and give the reader a glimpse of Drouart's embodied experience; after all, crossing borders was a complicated affair in eighteenth-century Europe. Burghart, living in Brieg, a town on the edges of the Prussian empire, appears impressed by Drouart's worldliness and use of German. Examining Drouart's body enabled Burghart to enter into dialogue with Mertrud, Morand, Vacherie, and Hoin, who were major figures in the European medical sphere. In the context of this "network of exchange" (Pomata, "Sharing Cases" 197), Burghart participated in the dialogue across national and linguistic boundaries that constructed Drouart as a "hermaphrodite" and himself as an established physician.

Burghart's title, *Gründliche Nachricht an seinen Freund *** Von einem neuerlich gesehenen Hermaphroditen, Wobey zugleich etwas von der Medicinischen Mode erwähnet wird* (1763) [Detailed report to his friend *** regarding a recently examined hermaphrodite, to which is added some discussion of medical fashion], suggests that the study of the "hermaphrodite" stands at the center of the treatise and that his reflections on medical fashions are merely appended. The twenty-four-page-long text itself, however, devotes only eight pages to Drouart, which follow rather than precede—as suggested by the title—Burghart's reflections on developments in the medical profession. In a manner similar to Parsons, Burghart embeds his empirical study in additional reflections about medicine. Burghart ridicules new types of medical training relating to empirical inquiries into the human body: "A few years at an institution of higher learning now create a real artist after the new fashion. A little bit of mathematics, a dissected human body, a few strangled dogs, some observed chemical experiments, an air pump that has been touched three times, and finally a bag full of metaphysical truths" ["ein paar Jahre Zeit auf der Hohen Schule bilden einen ächten Künstler nach der neuen Mode. Ein bißgen Mathematik, ein zerschnittner menschlicher Cörper, ein Paar erwürgte Hunde, etliche gesehene Chemische Versuche, eine dreimahl angerührte Lufftpumpe, und endlich ein Sackvoll metaphysischer Wahrheiten"] (5). For Burghart, the Drouart case serves as a platform from which to critique the eighteenth-century focus on empirical knowledge. Burghart's attempt to distance himself from "dissection artists" ["Zergliederungs-Künstler"] (22) is ambivalent, however, because he claims their usefulness when lamenting the fact that in cases of suspected "hermaphroditism" typically only the external genitals are dissected.

In conjunction with his critique of empirical knowledge gathering, Burghart also casts a critical look at one of its European centers, Paris. Burghart, who believes that Drouart is more likely to bear than to engender a child, considers the Sorbonne's judgment that Drouart was a man "ridiculous" ["lächerlich"] (21): "The Sorbonne was surprised by a report from a superstitious priest or a halfway intelligent surgeon, who are as common in Paris as they are at home, and transformed our Drouet from an obvious woman into a doubtful and frankly impossible man" ["die Sorbonne, durch, Gott weiss was vor einen elenden Bericht etwa eines abergläubischen Curé, oder eines halb klugen Wundarzts, die in Paris so wenig seltsam sein, als wie bei uns, überraschet worden, unsern Drouet aus einem offenbaren Mägden in eine sehr zweifelhafte, ja ganz unmögliche Mannsperson … zu verwandeln] (19–20). Burghart in particular critiques French surgical expertise when he describes the "Franzosen" as "great lovers of a fast and bold knife" ["grosse Liebhaber von einem hurtigen und verwegnen Messer"] (18). Burghart's ridiculing of the Sorbonne and French medical practice is embedded in a broader critique of the supremacy of French language, culture, and intellectual production in eighteenth-century Europe. Burghart mocks his contemporaries' infatuation with all things French: "We Germans and other nations are used to prize all things foreign and unusual, especially what is written to us from France" ["Wir Deutschen, und andre Nationen sind hernach gewohnet alles ausländische, und ungewöhnliche sehr hoch zu schätzen, insonderheit was sich aus Frankreich herschreibet"] (21). Burghart's fear of the feminizing effects of French culture and science dovetails with his comments regarding Drouart's questionable masculinity. Burghart, who describes himself as an old-fashioned physician, uses the Drouart case as a springboard for his commentary on developments in the medical sphere, which thinly veils his anxieties regarding his position in this changing context.

Burghart's 1763 critique of the French medical profession not only voices his own medical philosophy but also attempts to strengthen his position as a Prussian subject in Brieg, a town on the powerful state's periphery. Brieg had become part of Prussia twenty years earlier, in 1741, during the First Silesian War. Before that, it belonged to Austria. The fact that Burghart is writing in 1763 is significant in this context as that year marks the end of the Seven Years' War (1756–63), which opposed Britain and Prussia to France and Austria. By critiquing French medical education and French culture more generally, Burghart distances himself from the political opponent and aligns himself closely with the Prussian ruler Frederick II (the Great) and his militarization of the Prussian state. Burghart's dedication of the treatise to Frederick II was important in a context where institutions of medical instruction were closely connected to state power. Burghart presents himself as a loyal Prussian subject who has no allegiance to the Austrian-French coalition. In this respect, Burghart's insistence that Drouart should not be considered a man aligns with the Prussian construction of militarized masculinity. By ridiculing the Sorbonne's notion that Drouart was a man, Burghart echoed European perceptions of French men as weak and feminized, which allowed him to assert his loyalty to the Prussian state and consequently consolidate his professional standing in this context.

Heinrich Friedrich Delius, a German contemporary of Burghart who had trained at the universities of Berlin and Halle, was less suspicious of medical developments and French influence. He was serving as an anatomical demonstrator at the University of Erlangen-Nürnberg in 1765, when Drouart appeared on his doorstep during one of his lectures. Drouart enters the academic space of a German university and thereby provides Delius with an opportunity to engage Burghart's pamphlet directly. In contrast to Burghart, who thought of Drouart as a woman, Delius conceives of him as a "deformed man" ["eine verstaltete MannsPerson"] (404), in line with the Sorbonne's judgment. Delius also enters into dialogue with a specific issue mentioned by Burghart, namely the fact that only a postmortem autopsy would produce any new knowledge. Delius reports that Drouart "laughed and said that if he died here, he would gladly give permission to be dissected" ["mit Lachen sagte, daß wann er hier stürbe, er es [anatomisieren] gern erlauben wollte"] (404). As unsettling as this laugh may be, it expresses Drouart's profound understanding of the way in which medical professionals were using "hermaphrodite" bodies to strengthen their position. It is one of the few moments in which the "hermaphrodite's" subjectivity emerges, albeit, of course, mediated through the writing of the physician who presented the case and thereby ultimately controlled Drouart's representation.

The Hospital

Burghart's and Delius's discussion of the Sorbonne's medical assessment of Drouart shows the importance that universities and their affiliated hospitals began to play over the course of the eighteenth century. In German lands, especially in powerful states such as Prussia and Bavaria, medical authority resided in the hands of the government. As was the case in France, surgical knowledge gradually moved from the realm of apprenticeships to institutions of higher learning. In the German context, surgery was tied closely to universities, which were themselves connected to the court. Prussia in particular, where Burghart practiced and Delius was trained, inaugurated significant changes during the reign of Frederick William I (1688–1740), Frederick II the Great's father. Medicine had to be practical to improve the treatment of, first, the wounded on the battlefield and, second, the general population. In 1725, the collegium medico-chirurgicum was created so that doctors could be trained and examined in Prussia rather than abroad (Bleker and Hess 22); its creation institutionalized the teaching that happened at the theatrum anatomicum, which had been under the jurisdiction of the Academy of Sciences in Berlin since 1717. As Johanna Geyer-Kordesch observes, this meant that "surgeons were integrated with the 'learned' or university-based prestige of the internist" ("German Medical" 204).[24] From Berlin, the collegium medico-chirurgicum enforced its power throughout the state with the help of a network of regulations; it even shaped medical education in other states.

The consolidation of Prussian state authority can be seen in Frederick William I's establishment of a hospital for plague victims on the outskirts of Berlin in 1710. In 1724, with the gradual disappearance of the epidemic, the hospital changed its mission to become a treatment center for the sick poor; it was accordingly renamed the "Charité" and continued to train medical professionals, providing them with a steady stream of research subjects. In 1828, the Charité became the teaching hospital of the University of Berlin, which was founded in 1810, and exemplified the intertwinement of state power, medical training, and the university.

In 1801, Maria Dorothea Derrier, the 22-year-old daughter of poor laborers, arrived on the Charité's doorstep in search of treatment for scabies. In the process of giving their patient a therapeutic bath, physicians claimed to have discovered sexually ambiguous genitalia. The story of Derrier is closely tied to the emergence of professional medicine and the birth of the hospital as an institution for treating the sick and, eventually, as a research center in a rapidly growing metropolitan area. Developments in the British and French medical realm had already triggered reports on "hermaphrodites" earlier in the eighteenth and even the seventeenth century. It was only with the establishment of the Charité that Berlin became a contender in the European medico-scientific realm, rivaling Paris, London, Leiden, and Edinburgh.[25] When Derrier arrived in the Charité, the institution was well-established, even though it suffered from precarious financing and poor sanitary conditions. One of its specialties was the treatment of pregnant women and venereal diseases, especially in female prostitutes. As a poor woman suffering from scabies, a disease predominantly transmitted sexually, Maria Dorothea Derrier fit the profile of the typical Charité patient.

Medical Authorities and Newcomers

Over the course of a year, five case histories on Derrier were published by medical men whose professional standing illustrates the institutionalization of medicine, the rapprochement and eventual fusion of traditional academic medicine and surgery, and a growing critical stance toward these developments, not unlike that expressed earlier in the century by Burghart, in his commentary on the Drouart case. These histories were written not only by surgeons trying to establish themselves professionally but also by those medical men who were already part of the medical establishment and tried to maintain their relevance. Christoph Wilhelm Hufeland is a case in point. In 1801, the year that Derrier entered the Charité, Frederick William III appointed Hufeland as its director. Hufeland was one of the most famous eighteenth-century German physicians and had worked at the intellectual centers of Weimar and Jena. On the title page of his journal, the *Journal der practischen Arzneikunde und Wundarzneykunst* [Journal of practical pharmacology and surgery], in which he published his case history of Derrier, Hufeland emphasizes his institutional affiliation as the "royal Prussian privy, personal physician, director of the collegium medicum, chief physician at the Charité, etc" ["Königl. Preuss. Geheimen Rath, Leibarzt, Director des Colleg. med. chirurg., erstem Arzt der Charité, u.s.w."] (n.p.). At the same time that he underlines his connection to traditional academic medicine, Hufeland also aligns himself with surgical empiricism through the journal that he founded in 1795, the *Journal der practischen Arzneikunde und Wundarzneykunst.*-Emphasizing the practical aspect of medical knowledge positioned Hufeland strategically in the changing medical sphere. With his case history on Derrier, he claimed ownership of this discovery as the medical director of the Charité and thereby put "his" hospital on the map as a premiere research institution in the European realm, rivaling those in Britain and France.

In 1801, the same year, a second case history on Derrier was published by one of Hufeland's colleagues, Christian Ludwig Mursinna. In contrast to Hufeland, who was born into a family of renowned physicians, had studied at the universities of Jena and Göttingen, and treated such celebrities as Wieland, Herder, Goethe, Schiller, and King Friedrich Wilhelm III, Mursinna came to the medical profession from the tradition of barber-surgery and had therefore acquired his knowledge through an apprenticeship rather than an institution of higher learning (Gurlt 81–4). Mursinna had arrived in Berlin as an army surgeon and complemented his practical training by attending lectures and reading books on anatomy, physiology, and surgery. In 1775, he was appointed as the Charité's chief surgeon. His case history on Derrier, "Von einer besondern Naturbegebenheit," appeared in the inaugural issue of his own *Journal für die Chirurgie, Arzneykunde und Geburtshilfe* [Journal for surgery, pharmacology, and obstetrics]. Like the academically trained Hufeland, Mursinna—the barber-surgeon-turned-academic-physician—strategically published his study in a periodical that he had founded himself. By using the term "Chirurgie" ("surgery") rather than the older "Wundarzneikunst," which Hufeland still employed and which literally meant "the art of healing wounds," Mursinna emphasized surgery's gradual rise in status. Mursinna's study is six pages long and, although it does not reference Hufeland's comparatively short article explicitly, it expands on it implicitly by providing more detailed information on Derrier's genital anatomy both textually and visually in the appended illustrations. Mursinna repeatedly emphasizes that he personally viewed Derrier either by describing specific examination procedures or by relating conversations between himself and Derrier. Statements such as "after a more detailed examination" ["nach genauerer Untersuchung"] (556) and "I was able to insert the top of my little finger" ["ich konnte … die Spitze meines kleinen Fingers … hineinbringen"] (556) stand in sharp contrast to Hufeland, who exclusively uses the impersonal, third-person pronoun "man" ["one"] when describing the exam. Mursinna suggests that the Charité's director might not have been personally present at the exam and thereby obliquely ranks his own empirical credentials above those of Hufeland, who became his superior in 1801. Mursinna strives to remain deferential toward Hufeland, all the while asserting his own authority.

Hufeland's and Mursinna's publications reveal the medical fascination with "hermaphrodites." Other medical men, however, had a more critical stance toward the proliferation of these case histories in particular and developments in the medical profession more broadly. One such publication is "Von dem neuangekommenen Hermaphroditen in der Charité zu Berlin im Jahre 1801 und von Zwittern überhaupt" ["About the hermaphrodite who newly arrived in the Charité in 1801 and about hermaphrodites in general"] published in 1801, the same year as Hufeland's and Mursinna's journal articles. Like Mursinna, the author emphasizes that he saw Derrier firsthand and reveals that Derrier quickly became a medical attraction in the Charité, where "in addition to me, many others have already seen the hermaphrodite and continue their visits daily" ["ausser mir viele andere den Zwitter bereits schon gesehen haben, und noch täglich besuchen"] (6). The author's critical and even satirical stance surfaces in his choice of the pseudonym "Monorchis"; the adjective "monorchid" refers to a man with only one testicle. Monorchis questions the intense scrutiny of "hermaphrodites" when he sarcastically posits that "in the learned world, hermaphrodites multiply every day and will soon completely supplant the quiet lot of natural humans" ["das Zwittergeschlecht in der gelehrten Welt sich mit jedem Tage vermehrt, und bald das stille Häuflein von Naturmenschen gänzlich verdrängen wird"] (3). At the same time, however, he self-consciously reflects on the fact that he himself benefits from this discourse:

> It goes without saying that I, following the laudable custom of the authors of our time, cannot help but expand this small document with grand aesthetic-critical and natural-historical observations and excerpts and, in this way, introduce the chaste reader to the secrets of hermaphroditism. He will then be more prepared when he follows the way of all flesh to the Charité and shares his pros and cons with me.
>
> [Es versteht sich aber von selbst, daß ich nach der löblichen Gewohnheit der Schriftsteller des Tages nicht umhin kann, auch diese kleine Schrift mit großen ästhetisch-kritisch- und naturhistorischen Bemerkungen und Excerpten anzufüllen, und so den keuschen Leser in die Geheimnisse des Hermaphrodismus einzuweihen. Er wird alsdann desto vorbereiteter den Weg alles Fleisches nach der Charite finden, und sein Pro oder Contra mir mittheilen können.]. (3–4)

Monorchis points out the process at play in Parsons's text by which, despite eighteenth-century medicine's focus on empiricism, case histories on a single individual often ballooned because of excerpts and summaries from previously published writings. His satirical reference to the "chaste reader" also hints at these writings' voyeuristic dimension, which was, as the following chapters will show, central not only to their marketing but also to the creation of the category of the "hermaphrodite" in the first place. Monorchis's identity remains a mystery, yet his comments suggest that he was, or claimed to be, a physician at the Charité. Monorchis casts a critical-satirical look at the emerging position of Berlin as a medical center. By choosing a pseudonym that invokes a defect in masculinity, Monorchis not only mirrors the "hermaphrodite's" liminal identity but also pokes fun at the competitive masculinity of turn-of-the-century medical professionals and their jockeying for positions at prominent medical institutions.

Derrier became an unavoidable topic in the Berlin medical realm; even the most prominent physicians felt compelled to participate in the debate and thereby assert their intellectual weight. In 1801, Johann Christian Stark, dean of the medical college at Jena, opposed Hufeland, Mursinna, and Monorchis in his own journal, the *Neues Archiv für die Geburtshülfe, Frauenzimmer- und neugebohrner Kinderkrankheiten* [New archive for obstetrics and women's and infants' diseases]. After examining Derrier, Stark argued that, rather than being female, Derrier is "a deformed man" ["eine missgestaltete Mannsperson"] (551). With this conclusion, Stark opened the Derrier matter for further debate. This opportunity was seized by a less prominent physician, Franz Heinrich Martens, who, in 1802, published his own case history. Martens strategically negotiated the power dynamics of the eighteenth-century medical sphere by flattering Hufeland and Mursinna as "two famous men" ["zwei berühmte Männer"] (5) but aligning himself with Stark. This strategic move paid off professionally. Holding a doctorate from Jena and working as a physician in Leipzig, Martens, who was best known for his publication, *Versuch eines vollständigen Systems der theoretischen und praktischen Geburtshülfe* [Attempt at a complete system of theoretical and practical obstetrics], was promoted to a professorial position at Stark's hospital in Jena in 1804 (Winckel 460–1). Writing about "hermaphrodites" and entering into dialogue with other scientists presented opportunities as well as risks for these eighteenth-century physicians. As the following chapters will show, they rarely reflected on the ethical dimension of their investigations. Through their professional publications, eighteenth-century medical men asserted their own agency by erasing that of their research subjects.

Stark and Martens exemplify the fusion of traditional medical education—both were associated with the eminent university at Jena—and empirical medical knowledge at the turn of the century. This change is visible in the titles of the journals that they founded and edited. Martens's emphasis on the "theoretisch[e] und praktisch[e]" aspects of "Geburtshilfe," literally "birthing help," is most obvious in this respect. While for centuries the person assisting the woman giving birth had been a midwife, in the eighteenth century, men-midwives—physicians with surgical expertise and skilled in the use of the forceps—sought to establish a place for themselves in the birthing chamber. Even in the presence of these men, childbirth still largely took place in the confines of a private residence. However, the gradual institutionalization of medicine in university hospitals over the course of the eighteenth century prepared the shift of obstetrics from the private to a more public realm. This transition in turn provided further opportunities for physicians to gather empirical knowledge due to an influx of patients, initially from the lower social classes, which further increased the power differential in this medical encounter. In this respect, publications on "hermaphrodites" crystallize these developments and highlight the intersectional nature of identities with respect to gender, class, and ability.

Male physicians were increasingly consulted in cases of bodies that were considered to display nonstandard sexual anatomy at birth, which contributed to the erosion of midwives' authority. While male practitioners with direct experience of the female body used to occupy a liminal space in the medical sphere, as represented by Cruikshank's caricature of the man-midwife as a "hermaphrodite," they consolidated their professional standing over the course of the eighteenth century. Obstetrics gradually became a male profession. Publishing on "hermaphrodites" allowed these practitioners to be perceived less as "hermaphroditic" creatures themselves and more as respected members of the medical profession. In the German-language realm, periodical publications played an important role in establishing and consolidating physicians' professional identity, whereas in France the association to national and regional academies was more important. In Britain, the place where medical knowledge was the most commercialized, broadside-style publications promised the greatest rewards and notoriety.

At the same time that the Enlightenment portrayed empiricism as the ultimate mode of knowledge production, it already began to critique its premises and conclusions. The construction of the "hermaphrodite" illustrates this process in powerful ways. Eighteenth-century case histories of "hermaphrodites" typically lament that they are examining living bodies, which curtailed their information gathering. The reference to a possible autopsy of Drouart's body by Drouart himself acknowledges the high expectations attached to postmortem dissections. However, the case of Derrier shows that those whom Burghart and Monorchis satirically call "dissection artists" ["Zergliederungs-Künstler"] (Burghart 15, 17) and "dissectors" ["Zergliederer"] (Monorchis 14) were not able to resolve all ambiguities. In 1836, an autopsy of Derrier was performed by a Professor Mayer in Bonn; two accounts were published, one in the *Gazette Médicale de Paris* and the other in *The Lancet*.[26] *The Lancet* article concludes that male and female attributes are mixed to such a degree that it is impossible to decide on Derrier's sex: "On the one hand, a testicle, a penis, and a prostate; on the other hand, a uterus, with fallopian tubes, a vagina, and an ovary" ("Description of an Hermaphrodite" 142). Or, as the *Gazette Médicale* argues: "il peut exister de véritables hermaphrodites chez l'homme" ["there can be true hermaphrodites in humans"] ("Description Anatomique" 610). The autopsy, which had been thought to bring absolute certainty, does not put the Derrier matter to rest. And yet, autopsies continued to hold the promise of solving the mystery of "hermaphrodites." During the nineteenth century, which Alice Dreger has called the "Age of Gonads" (*Hermaphrodites* 11), the demonstrator in the anatomical theater would be replaced by the scientist in the laboratory peeking through the microscope and scrutinizing ovarian and testicular tissue in search of differentiating markers. Nineteenth-century dissection reports were directed at a specialized audience of medical professionals. The publications resulting from these autopsies were a sign of the increasing professionalization of medicine and the widening gap between academic medicine and more popular discourses on health. By contrast, eighteenth-century case histories still focused on living and breathing "hermaphrodites"; they thereby mirrored the increasingly popular genre of the novel, which also focused on the life story of an individual under extraordinary circumstances and thereby appealed to medical professionals and laypeople alike. The open-endedness of these case histories is a constitutive factor of eighteenth-century "hermaphrodite" ontology, which results in the publication of ever more case histories searching for definitive answers. These case histories reveal that the eighteenth-century confidence in the unambiguous truth of empirical facts was, after all, a fiction.

Notes

1 Cruikshank (1764–1811), a London-based Scottish painter and caricaturist, was best known for his satirical drawings of political and social issues.

2 The full title of Fores's treatise is *Man-Midwifery Dissected; or, the Obstetric Family Instructor for the Use of Both Sexes. Containing a Display of the Management of Every Class of Labour by Men and Boy Mid-Wives; also of Their Cunning, Indecent and Cruel Practices. Instructions to Husbands How to Counteract Them. A Plan for the CompleteInstruction of Women Who Possess Promising Talents, in Order to Supersede Malepractice. Various Arguments and Quotations, Proving, that Man-Midwifery Is a Personal, Domestic and a National Evil* (Wellcome Library).

3 Jean Towler and Joan Bramall describe how "gradually other titles came to be used [instead of 'man-midwife']. These included andro-boethygynist (man helper of

women), accoucheur (one who brings to childbed) and finally obstetrician, from the Latin obstetrix (to stand before)" (71).

4 The medical men of the English Chamberlen family are typically credited with the invention and popularization of the forceps (Towler and Bramall 77).

5 This process happened at different speeds in different contexts and was always contested by regular midwives. In the Anglo-Saxon context, described by Wilson, and Woods and Galley, the assertion of medical men in cases of normal births was stronger than in France, the German territories, the Dutch territories, or Spain (Wilson 5). See Lindemann, "Professionals," Robilliard, and Wiesner-Hanks, "The Midwives," on German-speaking territories. McTavish describes the process in early modern France. Also see Marland, and Towler and Bramall.

6 On the topic of female patients' social class, see Risse.

7 See Thomas on the complex process that established a midwife's credentials and the changing status of midwives in the early modern period.

8 As Adrian Wilson points out, they "were usually called 'surgeons,' rather than 'men-midwives,' and this tends to conceal their obstetric practice" (47).

9 In his *Emotions and Surgery*, which focuses on Romantic texts, Michael Brown has put "emotions back at the heart of the history of surgery" (3) by questioning the marginalization of emotions within surgical culture that, he argues, began in the second quarter of the nineteenth century, with the introduction of anesthesia and antisepsis techniques.

10 Susan Lawrence traces the gradual move of anatomical dissections from less to more respectable London neighborhoods, demonstrating surgeons' gradual increase in respectability. Clifford Morgan provides a detailed discussion of the surgical profession and a number of prominent surgeons in eighteenth-century London.

11 Depending on the context, this process occurred at different moments. In France, a series of royal edicts resulted in the creation of the Academy of Surgery in 1731. In Prussia, a 1725 edict led to the establishment of the *collegium medico-chirurgicum*. In England, the surgeons separated from the barbers in 1745 and founded the Company of Surgeons. In addition to Bonner on this topic, also see Brockliss and Jones, Brown (*Performing Medicine*), Gelfand, Geyer-Kordesch, "Court Physician" and "German Medical Education," Porter (*The Greatest Benefit*), and Spary, "Health."

12 See Bonner on the national and regional differences in the eighteenth-century European medical realm.

13 In London's entrepreneurial setting, Douglas was one of the first medical professionals to teach a public course on anatomy (Guerrini 172–3). In recognition of his professional standing, the Royal Society appointed Douglas as its anatomical demonstrator.

14 Brian McInnis surveys the process by which empirical science gradually replaced older forms of knowledge production and the resulting tensions and contradictions.

15 For a discussion of the origin and development of the concept of a vitalistic life force, "Lebenskraft," see McCarthy et al.

16 All translations are mine, unless otherwise noted.

17 In his 1788 compilation of famous trials, Nicolas-Toussaint des Essarts highlights Grandjean's humble provenance: "Grandjean étoit un esprit fort simple, qui avoit reçu dans la maison de son père une education grossière & laborieuse … une existence pauvre" ["Grandjean had a very simple mind and had received a coarse education focused on manual labor in his father's house … a poor existence"] (122).

18 Socially and economically disadvantaged individuals, both domestic and colonial, would become research subjects in medical experiments in the eighteenth century. On this topic, see Schiebinger, "Human Experimentation." Chapter 4 of *Medicalizing Difference* discusses the alignment of poor domestic subjects with those from Britain's colonies.

19 For full titles, see the "Primary Texts" section in Works Cited.

20 For a discussion of entries on "hermaphrodites" in eighteenth-century reference works, and the *Encyclopédie* in specific, see Hilger, "Orientation."

21 A discussion of the way in which medical practitioners positioned themselves in the medical print market in England can be found in Blackwood and Williams, Fissell, and Furdell.

22 The history of the *Jardin du Roi* as an institution of natural history and medical training is described in Spary, *Utopia's Garden*.

23 For an account of the pamphlet warfare between physicians and surgeons, also see Gelfand 58–79.

24 Geyer-Kordesch provides a detailed account of the complex relationship between the collegium medico-chirurgicum and the theatrum anatomicum ("German Medical"). The emergence of medical science in eighteenth-century Prussia is also discussed in Geyer-Kordesch's "Court Physician and State Regulation."

25 For a history of the Charité, see Bleker and Hess, Einhäupl, and Jaeckel.

26 While neither publication was written by Mayer himself, both report his observations.

2

Entertainment Science

Publishing a case history on a "hermaphrodite" was a way for eighteenth-century physicians to establish and strengthen their position in a rapidly changing medical sphere, to the detriment of their object of study who was medicalized and pathologized through a discourse that fused empiricism with new publishing conventions. Even the most famous and respected medical men felt the necessity to publicize their professional qualifications, as the example of Christoph Wilhelm Hufeland shows. Despite his prominent position as the Weimar court physician, Hufeland was never secure financially and had to generate supplemental revenue by giving lectures to fee-paying students in Jena. Becoming the director of the premiere teaching hospital in Berlin, the Charité, provided Hufeland with a more stable income.[1] In this context, publishing a case history on Maria Dorothea Derrier in 1801 in his own journal, *Journal der practischen Arzneikunde und Wundarzneykunst*, was a strategic move that served a number of intertwined purposes. It enabled Hufeland to claim ownership of this discovery, publicize his professional credentials, and position his hospital as one of the premiere research institutions in the European medical realm.

Hufeland's approach toward the topic of "hermaphroditism" mirrors that of his contemporaries. Authors actively publicized their case histories; they thereby reacted to the gradual commercialization of the medical sphere, yet they also questioned this development. The more closely these medical men were tied to an academic medical background, the more ambivalent they felt toward these changes, not least because they feared that commodifying their knowledge would undermine their reputation. Conversely, those who came from a nontraditional background, such as barber surgeons, also felt unsure about these developments. Their ambivalence, however, stemmed from their status as the new arrivals in a sphere still dominated by their academic colleagues, who continued to be held in higher esteem.

Medical Collections and Journals

Medical journalism flourished in the eighteenth century (Kronick, "Medical" 277–82). In the earlier part of the century, it took the form of contributions to the collections of national and regional academies: Morand published his study in *Mémoires de l'Académie Royale des Sciences de Paris*, Hoin in *Mémoires de l'Académie de Dijon*, Ferrein in *Histoire de l'Académie Royale*, and Delius in *Fränkische Sammlungen von Anmerkungen aus der Naturlehre*. Placing their case histories in the publications of reputable professional associations conferred respectability and trustworthiness to these authors. Over the course of the century, however, a new type of periodical emerged that gained in popularity alongside these more traditional collections: the medical journal.[2] In contrast to present-day academic medical periodicals, the editor often was also the journal's founder and most of the contributions were written by the editors themselves, as Hufeland's example demonstrates. Hufeland was not the only one who authored a case history and published it in his own journal, so did Stark and Mursinna. Like the collections of national and regional academies, these journals served to establish the professional standing of their editors and authors, two entities that overlapped frequently, but they did so from a more entrepreneurial vantage point. Medical journals served as an advertising platform that allowed their authors/editors to publicize their expertise and services, not only to the medical community but also to the general population. As Laurence Brockliss and Collin Jones observe, "Although clearly aimed at fellow-practitioners, none of these medical journals closed themselves off from the general reader" (647). Scientific knowledge in the eighteenth century was becoming increasingly popularized and was marketed to a growing reading public, to whom the "hermaphrodite" was marketed both as a natural curiosity and an object of entertainment.

Natural History Bestsellers

Case histories on "hermaphrodites" were part of the broader popularization of writings on natural history, published in the vernacular rather than in Latin. Many books in this genre became bestsellers because they appealed to a broad audience. Monorchis, author of a case history on Derrier, references the public's voracious consumption of these publications when he observes that the "printed descriptions are sold out and devoured" ["Die gedruckten Beschreibungen werden vergriffen und verschlungen"'] (3). In addition to articles in medical journals and in the collections of medical societies, some case histories appeared as independent publications. While there were elaborately produced case histories with intricate artwork that only a well-read and well-heeled elite could afford,[3] other formats also existed such as broadsides, which were not only affordable but also geared at readers with limited literacy. These broadside-style texts, such as those by Vacherie and Martens, typically did not exceed twenty pages.[4] Even a full-length book such as James Parsons's *Enquiry* was within reach for many as it cost "three shillings and sixpence, almost the same price as the exhibition of the African" (Fontes da Costa 132–3). Those who had not been able to see the exhibit of the Angolan "hermaphrodite" in London could recreate the experience by purchasing Parsons's text.

The increasing number of publications on natural history was a function of the overall growth of the book market, which was itself closely connected to the rise in literacy rates over the course of the eighteenth century. While definitions of literacy during this period vary—ranging from the competence to sign one's name on a legal document to the ability to read an entire novel—there is no doubt that an increasing number of people could read, partly due to reforms in national and regional schooling systems and that the publishing realm catered to the demands of this growing audience.[5] In the wake of the Reformation, the capacity to read the Bible directly was the motor for acquiring literacy, and consequently religious publications dominated the book market. In the second half of the eighteenth century, however, the proportion of religious and nonreligious books changed dramatically. Reading for entertainment established itself as a practice and resulted in a steep increase in published material of a nonreligious nature.[6] Popularized medical case histories on "hermaphrodites" were strategically positioned in the realm where science and the novel met, resulting in a specifically eighteenth-century form of entertainment science

Erotic Empiricism

Science's empirical focus on living creatures, often those with unusual physiological traits, was mirrored by the genre of the novel, which emerged and became extremely popular over the course of the eighteenth century.[7] Fiction portrayed the story of an individual, often living in unusual or extreme circumstances. Like natural history, it extensively described the individual's appearance and detailed the experience of existing in a difficult and often hostile environment. In this respect, as Jason Tougaw has argued, the "case history is the British novel's most influential analogue … In the pages of a medical journal, the quest for knowledge is entangled with the need to tell a good story; in the pages of a novel, appeals to a reader's sympathy first require characters whose flaws, or diagnoses, are severe enough to deserve it" (2). "Good stories" were those that elicited the reader's sympathy by portraying individuals who were subject to mistreatment by powerful individuals in their surroundings. In this respect, the struggles of "hermaphrodites" mirror those of the best-known protagonists, often female, of the eighteenth century. Their bodies and their sexuality stand at the center of a text that purports a specific purpose—empirical knowledge gathering and moral instruction—yet undermines it through its voyeuristic dimension. The readers' investment in these stories resulted in additional writings, either in the form of new case histories or sequels, which blurred the line between historical and fictional characters and between science and entertainment at the same time that they sought to consolidate this separation.

One of the most popular novels of the period was Samuel Richardson's *Pamela; or, Virtue Rewarded.* First published in 1740, the novel quickly became a bestseller and was widely translated and imitated. *Pamela* was the model for a genre in which a young woman, typically a bourgeois virgin, was in danger of being morally corrupted by a more experienced man, often an aristocratic rogue. The French and the German literary traditions adapted this genre, which became as famous on the continent as it was across the channel. Richardson's *Pamela*, Sophie von LaRoche's *Die Geschichte des Fräulein von Sternheim* (1771), and Julie de Krüdener's *Valérie* (1803) were a version of conduct literature for young women, warning them about the dangers of physical seduction and moral corruption. Each text presented a heterosexual ending, in which the protagonist either consented to the male protagonist's advances or was coerced by him. In this respect, Paul Kelleher describes these novels as an "aggressively normalizing fiction—sentimental heterosexuality" (197) that, through the "heterosexualization of moral sentiment … produced a new form of subjectivity" (19) and conflated "sexual desire and moral sensibility" (99).

Despite authors' assertions to the contrary, the voyeuristic aspect of novels à la *Pamela* aligned them with eighteenth-century pornographic literature, the origins of which lay in French libertine fiction, which combined the depiction of sexual encounters with political criticism. Pornography became the logical extension of novels such as *Pamela*, as Lynn Hunt argues: "Pornography engaged the same paradoxes of imagination and reality as the novel, and novels were also regularly condemned for their capacity to incite desire. Some pornography, then, is simply a specialized version of the novel; it plays upon the imagination of the reader to create the effect of real sexual activity, all the while, of course, being purely imaginary" (Hunt 37).[8] Hunt contends that "Sade parodied the interminable scenes of seduction found in novels such as Richardson's *Pamela*" (37). In contrast to Richardson, in the fiction of the Marquis de Sade, one of the most prominent authors of libertine/pornographic novels, the seduction scenes lead to minute and graphic descriptions of sexual encounters. Kathleen Lubey describes the space where sentimental fiction and pornography intersect as "eroticism," which she defines as "a literary mode collectively established by disparate texts, often episodically, as they experiment with formal and thematic strategies for describing sex that remain connected to some more epistemological purpose" (29). The stated goal of both types of texts was the moral instruction of readers who were invited to reflect on the protagonists' behavior in the middle of erotic descriptions and thereby to learn about their own moral character.

The eighteenth-century novel was predicated on the notion that self-knowledge could be achieved by observing others and reflecting on their actions, including the reactions of their body. Aileen Douglas argues that "novels, because they minutely register the perpetual and diverse affects of body upon body, insinuate that the predicaments of human physicality are at the heart of most stories" (xvi). Fictional protagonists therefore functioned as "scientific specimens" (xiv), especially in the epistolary genre, which conveyed an air of authenticity to the narrated events concerning fictional individuals and their bodies. Case histories on "hermaphrodites," which promised revelations about their subject's anatomy and behavior, appealed to the same type of voyeurism as Richardson's and Sade's novels. These narratives align the "hermaphroditic" body—and its threat to reproductive heterosexuality—with disabled bodies. This alignment is significant because, as Jason Farr argues, during this period, "impaired bodies are thus fundamental to the cultural construction of homo- and heterosexuality" (1). Eighteenth-century authors thereby "expose able-bodiedness and heterosexuality as imbricated systems that sustain dominant models of reproductive futurity" (1).

Authors strove to position their detailed investigations of a "hermaphrodite's" reproductive organs in a purely scientific realm, yet developments in the publishing realm had created multiple intersections between academic and popular writing, the medical case history and fiction, especially of the epistolary kind. In addition to the voyeurism inherent in both types of texts, they also shared the same empirical approach. In *The Experimental Imagination*, a study of literary knowledge and science in the British Enlightenment, Tita Chico comments on the popularization and inclusion of scientific empiricism in eighteenth-century narrative. Similarly, Helen Thompson, exploring the intersections between science and fiction, argues that "eighteenth-century novels make explicit the *production* of sensational understanding as the reader's encounter with forms and powers that enable empirical knowledge" (17; emphasis in original). The production of empirical knowledge is predicated on a voyeuristic form of power that implicates author and reader. As a result, "scientific examination could not be easily separated from the prurient curiosity of popular entertainment and erotic objectification" (Gilbert 136–7) and the "writers of medical and paramedical enquiries into hermaphrodites skillfully manipulated the slippage between these unstable terms" (142).[9] Case histories on "hermaphrodites" became a genre in its own right, with its own conventions, narrative structures, and tropes, which resulted from the interplay of scientific writings with other discourses such as the novel. In both of these genres, the narrator's empiricism—the minute investigation into the protagonists' bodies and their reactions—imbues these texts with a voyeuristic dimension that was predicated on the erasure of the main character's agency.

Empirical Voyeurism

The intertwinement of empiricism and erotic/pornographic voyeurism surfaces in the case histories' titles. The titles typically emphasize the firsthand examination of the "hermaphrodite's" body, sometimes with a geographical reference that grounds the author in his scientific and intellectual context. The scientists' active role rests on the "hermaphrodite's" passive position, grammatically represented by the passive voice: "about a recently *seen* hermaphrodite" ["von einem neuerlich *gesehenen* Hermaphroditen"] (Burghart; emphasis added), "*observed* hermaphrodite in Berlin" ["zu Berlin *beobachteten* weiblichen Hermaphroditen"] (Hufeland; emphasis added), "that has *appeared* before the eyes of the public" ["qui a *paru* aux yeux du public"] (Mertrud, emphasis added), and "that was *seen* in Paris" ["que l'on *voyait* à Paris"] (Morand, "Description d'un hermaphrodite," emphasis added). Some case histories use this firsthand visual examination inductively, to comment on "hermaphroditism" in general: "about hermaphrodites in general" ["und von Zwittern überhaupt"] (Monorchis) and "reflections on hermaphrodites" ["Réflexions sur les Hermaphrodites"] (Champeaux). Other histories muse on the medical profession at large by addressing developments in "medical fashion" ["von der medizinischen Mode"] (Burghart). For the audience, the title's emphasis on the visual inspection served as a voyeuristic preview of the content, thereby further blurring the line between science and entertainment at both the textual and the visual level.

Vacherie's broadside-style title functions as a summary of the contents and caters to the eighteenth-century public's desire for salacious reading material: "An Account of the Famous Hermaphrodite, or, Parisian Boy-Girl, Aged Sixteen, Named Michael-Anne Drouart, at This Time (November, 1750) upon Show in Carnaby-Street, London. With its Portrait Engraved from the Life." Vacherie's characterization of Drouart as a "boy-girl" blurs the line between scientific and erotic/pornographic literature. His use of the pronoun "it" signals Drouart's nonbinary sex and projects Drouart into a space of less-than-human abjection, which is reinforced by the voyeuristic description of Drouart's external genitals: "These Nymphae appear comparatively small and inconsiderable, though they so far agree with those in Virgins, that they are so firm, hard and solid" (10). In contrast to Vacherie's graphic explicitness, Monorchis, in his treatise on Derrier, uses an ellipsis: "Decency does not allow me to say more" ["Mehr erlaubt mir die Decenz nicht zu sagen"] (5). Monorchis's stated goal is to protect the "chaste reader" ["keuschen Leser"] (4) from such explicit material, yet his omission titillates the audience's curiosity even further. While Vacherie's explicit descriptions echo the graphic nature of the period's pornographic novels, the restraint displayed by Monorchis was common in sentimental fiction such as *Pamela* (1740). In both types of fiction, the threat of rape causes narrative suspense. In *Pamela*, the eponymous protagonist's master, Mr. B., repeatedly attempts to violate Pamela but does not succeed. In one particularly graphic description, he searches for letters exchanged between Pamela and her family and friends:

> "I have searched every place above, and in your closet, for them, and can't find them … it is my opinion they are about you; and I never undressed a girl in my life; but I will now begin to strip my pretty Pamela" … And he began to unpin my handkerchief. I wept, and resisting said, "I will not be used in this manner. Pray, sir, consider!" "And, pray," said he, "do *you* consider. For I *will* see these papers. But, perhaps," said the wicked wretch, (was ever any one so vile!) "they are tied about your knees with you garters;" and stooped. I fell on my knees, excessively affrighted." (271; emphasis in original)

Mr. B's desire to know Pamela's thoughts and actions—as recorded in her letters—translates into his violent attack of her body. His physical encroachment, represented by his removal of Pamela's outer items of clothing and his threat to proceed to her undergarments, mirrors the narrative structure in case histories on "hermaphrodites:" the physician is the powerful male who threatens his subject with his probing fingers in the quest to uncover the body's secret text. In his case history, for example, Hoin provides a detailed account of his intrusive physical examination of Drouart who is being described as

> very sensitive when the probe is introduced; ordinarily even a few droplets of blood emerge … We inserted a bougie until the hermaphrodite felt some painful pressure and we were not able to push it any further: it had been pressed in more than four inches.
>
> [fort sensible au moment de l'introduction de la sonde; elle fait même ordinairement sortir quelques gouttelettes de sang … Nous y avons fait pénétrer une bougie, jusqu'a ce que l'Hermaphrodite ressentit une légère impression douloureuse, & qu'il ne nous fut pas possible de la pousser plus avant: elle étoit enfoncée de plus de quatre pouces.] (5)

Drouart's pain and the violence wielded by the examiner parallel the power differential in the scenes of eighteenth-century novels focusing on a virtuous young woman' struggles to defend her virginity. In case histories, however, these voyeuristic descriptions are legitimized with the language of scientific empiricism and medical professionalism. These detailed and often lengthy accounts are predicated on the availability of subaltern individuals whose bodies were medicalized through the language of entertainment science. A close reading of this language uncovers the authors' ideological investment in the pathologization of individuals with variable sex characteristics and thereby serves to denaturalize their construction as "hermaphrodites."

Double entendres permeate the language of entertainment science and further contribute to the porno-scientific tone typical for the eighteenth-century case history. Parsons's *Mechanical and Critical Enquiry* (1741) abounds with this type of word play, even though its title strives to position the treatise in the purely scientific realm. At the end of his introduction, after a reference to the Angolan and his explanation of the term *Macroclitorideus*, Parsons states that his goal is to "reduc[e] the Matter to a Certainty" (liv). In a scientific treatise that focuses on disproportionally large clitorises, comments such as "a small difference in a word makes a great variation in the idea that should be proportioned to the thing treated of" (96) cement the text's salacious undercurrent. When Parsons refers to the "divided scrotum of certain authors" (82) and describes their "hermaphrodital affair" (83), he teases the reader with the promise of scandalous revelations. He further comments that his review of previous literature on the topic of human "hermaphroditism" caused his text to "swell … to its present size" (v) but was necessary to trace the "erection" (9) of these authors' theories. In a work on individuals that were considered to have nonstandard sexual anatomy, such turns of phrase are neither coincidental nor innocent as they indicate the permeable and shifting boundary between scientific and erotic/pornographic literature. The ontology of the "hermaphrodite" is inextricably intertwined with the capitalist logic of the eighteenth-century publishing marketplace. The absence of any ethical reflections in these authors' case histories constructs "hermaphrodite" subjects as liminal bodies without any regard for their embodied experience.

Illustrations

The conventions of scientific discourse and erotic/pornographic literature also intersect in the illustrations that accompany most of the published case histories.[10] These visual renderings are typically advertised on the title page—Vacherie highlights the "portrait engraved from the life" —and range in quality, from amateurish drawings to professional artwork. Martens, for example, calls existing illustrations of Derrier "pitiful" ["erbärmlich"] (5) and thus justifies writing his own case history and illustrating it himself: "I drew the attached copperplates to represent nature and I believe I can flatter myself that the imitation is rather faithful" ["Ich zeichnete die beigefügten Kupfertafeln nach der Natur, und ich glaube, mir schmeicheln zu dürfen, daß die Nachahmung ziemlich treu sein möchte"] (12). Others, like Stark, do not include a visual rendering but feel the need to address this lacuna: "A drawing might have made the description clearer but I did not have enough time" ["Eine Zeichnung davon würde vielleicht die Beschreibung anschaulicher machen, aber die Zeit war mir zu kurz"] (551). Stark's urgency to usher his case history into print serves as an excuse for omitting the type of illustration that readers had come to expect by the turn of the century.

Illustrations, which were central to eighteenth-century erotic/pornographic literature, thereby became part of the conventions of the "hermaphrodite" case history genre. While some authors, like Martens, drew the "hermaphrodite's" genitals themselves, others included illustrations produced by professionals, as was the case with Drouart. In fact, Drouart's "fame" started not with a published case history but with a piece of art, which is mentioned by Vacherie: "Sieur Gautier, a celebrated Engraver, painted and graved a Portrait of it … which he had the Honour to present to the King of *France*, who received it so graciously as to appoint him a pension" (5; emphasis in original; also in Courtney Thompson 398). Gautier d'Agoty was a French anatomist, painter, and printmaker who was best known for his production of colorful and lavish anatomical illustrations. His painting of Drouart, not included in Vacherie's cheap pamphlet, was originally produced to accompany Mertrud's case history; it was also published in d'Agoty's own *Observations sur l'histoire naturelle* in 1752 and subsequently reprinted in his *Collection de planches d'histoire naturelle* in 1757. Mertrud, the king's surgeon and royal anatomical demonstrator, had commissioned the painting and by doing so had secured the artist's livelihood. Vacherie points out that by the time he published his own study, "this print is at this Time grown pretty rare" (5), attesting to the popularity of visual material regarding the "hermaphrodite." The "hermaphrodite" served as a means for artists to make a foray into the field of anatomical illustrations, which was to become increasingly profitable as it was, like case histories, situated in the field of entertainment science.

The most elaborate illustrations can be found in James Parsons's *Enquiry*. The largest of those is a foldout reproduction of an illustration of the genitals of the Angolan and of another, unidentified female by Dr. James Douglas, whom Parsons assisted in his anatomical studies. Then, there are two regular-size plates. The first of those is an engraving of the Angolan's genitals, which is meant to supplement Douglas's drawing. The second one presents the dissected genitals of the female fetus referenced in Parsons's preface. The foldout illustration is not only the largest but also the most spectacular of the three plates because it presents three genital areas as if they were part of one single body. Only the captions make it clear that these genitals do not belong to one single individual. The first genital area on this plate is that of the Angolan "hermaphrodite" and the other two are illustrations of the genitals of another woman, the first with the labia closed, the second with the labia opened. Showing the closed alongside the opened labia portrays the empirical process of the male scientist who explores the dark mystery of the "hermaphrodite," catering to his readers' voyeuristic desires. As Courtney Thompson argues, "Visual depictions of hermaphrodites … were caught between practices of scientific, artistic, and pornographic illustration" (393). In Parsons's text, the scientific genre intersects not only with pornographic literature but also with travelogues about remote places; his *Enquiry* therefore echoes the discursive conventions of what Anne McClintock has called "the porno-tropic" (22). The foldout bears resemblance to a landscape with craters, hills, ridges, and forests that, in its mystery and opaqueness, calls for investigation and exploration.

This illustration functions in a manner similar to, what Darby Lewes has called "somatopias" in early modern pornographic literature which present "women's bodies (or more accurately, a generalized female body) as a site of male pleasure: a utopian sexual landscape" (167). One subtype of the somatopia, the imperial somatopia, "depict[s] women as foreign lands … in need of conquering" (167). In this sense, "hermaphroditic" bodies become the last frontier in the scientist's quest to understand and thereby control uncharted territory, as will be shown in detail in Chapter 4.

Ambivalence

Even though medical professionals were actively involved in the book market for entertainment science, they felt ambivalent about their role in it, not because of any ethical qualms but because of fears regarding their professional reputation. On the one hand, market forces compelled them to advertise their expertise and services. On the other, however, physicians and scientists worried that their participation in this consumer culture would cast doubt on their qualifications and reputation. As Chapter 1 has shown, one of the strategies used by medical men to navigate this situation was to highlight their professional affiliations and any connections to powerful contemporaries, either on the title page or in the text. Burghart's emphasis on his connections is the most extensive one; he devotes seven pages of his treatise to a dedication to the Prussian king and includes the exhortation: "Love me constantly" ["Lieben Sie mich beständig"] (24). Despite authors' strategic self-positioning in their case histories' preliminary pages, ambivalence regarding their participation in entertainment science continues to permeate their texts. Parsons, for example, explicitly reflects on the fact that his treatise has a double audience, laypeople and medical professionals. He directly addresses the Royal Society, of which he was a fellow and to whose members he had previously presented his research on a "hermaphroditic" fetus. He expresses his awareness that "some, perhaps, may ask what I have said in this Treatise, that they did not already know?" (v). He posits that his reason for writing is to dispel the "superstitious Mysteries and Errors" (vi) held not by his colleagues but by the general public, which gives him the opportunity to summarize and translate previous treatises on the topic of human "hermaphroditism." Parson's goal is to demonstrate that eighteenth-century science is in the process of dispelling all previous myths. However, producing an encyclopedic reader's digest that extensively excerpts and "ma[kes] English" (vii) those same myths—rather than merely recording his own empirical research—contributes to their persistence in the popular imagination. Providing the reader with these fantastical accounts in an affordable publication serves as a strategic marketing tool by "blurring distinctions between specialist interests and the curiosity of non-experts" (Stephanson and Wagner 9).

One particularly telling example of Parsons's simultaneous denial and reaffirmation of earlier sensationalist accounts is his presentation of the writings of Isbrand van Diemerbroeck, a seventeenth-century Dutch physician and anatomist. He offers gratuitous excerpts from Diemerbroeck's text, with a double entendre, "for the Reader's satisfaction" (126): "'Lately a Woman of no little Credit complained to me, that in her younger Days, having early Desires, she often rubbed that Part (the Clitoris) with her Finger, so as to provoke the Emission of Semen with much Delight, and that in some time this ill Custom caused it to become a Disease'" (127). Parsons's English translation of Diemerbroeck's text, the original Latin of which is presented in a footnote, highlights the close connection between capitalism, empiricism, and erotic/pornographic voyeurism in the eighteenth-century publishing realm geared toward "all Lovers of Truth in Natural History" (liv). Parsons is not the only author to summarize such accounts, some of which stem from Antiquity. Most of the authors, except for Vacherie and Delius, do so as well, albeit to varying degrees, pointing at the revenue potentials of these types of readers' digests that condense mythological accounts of "hermaphrodites" in a way that aligns them with the period's erotic and pornographic fiction.

The Lost Voice of the "Hermaphrodite"

Medical men's professional status was predicated on the erasure of the "hermaphrodites," whose voices are lost in the documents of the time. As subalterns, they were typically socially and economically dispossessed and often illiterate. They were therefore de facto excluded from the sphere in which those who created them as a category of medical discourse operated.[11] In that void, others established themselves, such as the lawyer Vermeil, who wrote in defense of Grandjean. His publication both mirrored and contributed to the "opinion publique" (9) after Grandjean's original condemnation for having lived as a man: "The news had been seized avidly by the public and was already spreading from mouth to mouth" ["la nouvelle avoit été saisie avec avidité par le Public & voloit déjà de bouche en bouche"] (8). By exhorting the reader to sympathize with Grandjean, Vermeil presents himself as a defender of Grandjean, who does not have a voice, and thereby opposes medical authorities: "It is in the secret of the narrowest prison and in the most horrible solitude that he devours his pain" ["C'est dans le secret de la prison la plus étroite, & et réduit à la plus affreuse solitude, qu'il dévore la douleur"] (9). At the same time that Vermeil presents himself as Grandjean's advocate—the French "avocat" means "lawyer"—he, like those who shaped Grandjean's story before him, profits financially from Grandjean's predicament, through the publication of his own pamphlet.

Vermeil was not the only one who appealed to the reader's sympathy by attempting to speak *for* Grandjean. A poem that appeared in 1765, the same year as Vermeil's *Mémoire*, pursued the same goal: *L'Hermaphrodite, ou Lettre de Grandjean à Françoise Lambert, sa femme*. The poem purports to be an authentic letter from Grandjean to their wife, yet it was actually written by

Edouard-Thomas Simon, a physician-turned-author.[12] In ten pages of rhymed verse, the narrator, supposedly Grandjean himself, laments their fate, arguing that a jealous rival is at the origin of the lawsuit. Grandjean describes their daily routine with their wife, invokes nature and God, and underlines their ignorance about their anatomical condition:

> They pursue the crime and I am innocent …
> What! I am in their shackles! … It is I … Terrible moment!
> Why? What have I done? O heavens! Is it possible? …
> I am nothing but a monster, a bizarre composite,
> A horrible and rare example of the play of nature …
> I have to be separated from the one that I adore.
> Law imposes a powerful judgment on me …
> What the eternal one has made, man dares to unmake… our bonds are holy…
> O barbarous nature! Your instinct joins us and your law separates us.
>
> [Ils poursuivent le crime, & je suis innocent ….
> Quoi! Je suis dans leurs fers! … C'est moi …. Moment terrible!
> Pouquoi? Qu'ai-je donc fait? O Ciel! Est-il possible? …
> Je ne suis plus qu'un monstre, un composé bizarre,
> Des jeux de la Nature exemple affreux & rare ….
> Il faut me séparer de celle que j'adore.
> Un Arrêt tout puissant m'en impose la Loi….
> Ce qu'a fait l'Éternel, l'homme ose le défaire…. nos liens sont sacrés….
> O Nature barbare! Ton instinct nous unit & ta Loi nous sépare.] (10–15)

The poem references the fact that, even though Grandjean was the protagonist of medical and legal case histories, they did not write these narratives. Literally and metaphorically shackled, Grandjean was unable to shape their representation and provide a counternarrative to the medical reports in which they appear as a "bizarre composite" and even a "monster." With his poem, Simon attempted to imagine Grandjean's embodied experience and subjectivity, which had been by erased by the medical case histories that scientists and laypeople alike devoured. Even though he was a physician himself, Simon presents himself as a counterweight to the medical men who focused exclusively on Grandjean's body to the detriment of their embodied experience. At the same time, however, his publication positions himself in the same market for entertainment science as the physicians whom he criticized. As an independent publication, his *Lettre de Grandjean* explored the revenue potential of this topic, while shaping public opinion by speaking for the person who, because of their social status and position as an object of medical research, had no voice.

Simon was not the only writer who positioned himself in this ambivalent way. In his 1788 account of famous eighteenth-century court cases, *Procès fameux*, Nicolas-Toussaint des Essarts also imagines Grandjean's perspective by giving them a fictional voice: " 'Today (said the unfortunate one to the magistrates of parliament) that my eyes have been opened to my fate, am I not miserable enough existing, without having the arm of justice striking me down? I was thrown onto the earth by accident, condemned to live in solitude' " [" 'Aujourd'hui (disoit cet infortuné aux magistrats du parlement) que mes yeux sont ouverts sur mon sort, ne suis je pas assez malheureux de me connoître sans que le bras de la justice s'appesantisse sur moi? Individu jetté comme hasard sur la terre, condamné à vivre dans la solitude' "] (124–5). Des Essarts uses quotation marks to indicate that he is recording Grandjean's direct speech. It is unclear, however, whether these are the historical Grandjean's exact words; in fact, large parts of Grandjean's speech here resemble Simon's poem. What is authentic about them, however, is the desire to generate sympathy in the reader by imagining the voice of the silenced Grandjean. In turn, the appeal to the reader's compassion is embedded in Des Essarts's awareness of the need to include the Grandjean case in his collection of famous court cases to increase its circulation and consequently his revenue and reputation.

(Un)Ethics

The "hermaphrodite's" lack of agency is an issue that not only shapes but renders possible all eighteenth-century case histories, yet it is never addressed directly. Authors do not explicitly thematize the ethical dimension of the professional and financial benefit they gained from the "hermaphrodite's" predicament. However, their awareness of their complicity surfaces in various guises. In Vacherie's text, it takes the shape of a detailed explanation of the economic factors transforming Drouart from a private citizen into a public figure. Vacherie explains that a surgeon took in Drouart, the child of working-class parents who had several other children to support, and exhibited Drouart for the fee of "thirty Louis-d'ors per Diem" (6). Vacherie also mentions that the painter Gautier d'Agoty produced an illustration that provided him with a royal "pension of six hundred Livres per annum" (5). Vacherie's unease surfaces when he provides apologetic explanations for the surgeon's and the painter's involvement. He explains that Drouart's parents were "not very easy in their circumstances" (5), that the surgeon "admitted but Persons of the first Rank and Condition" (6), and that d'Agoty "now actually enjoys" (5) his pension, implying that this was not the case initially, for unspecified reasons. These comments appear as displaced justifications for Vacherie's own participation in the marketing of Drouart's story. His stated reason for producing his pamphlet is to democratize scientific knowledge by addressing the "numbers of Persons who probably may never have an Opportunity of a personal Visitation" (6). As the author of a broadside publication that generated direct revenue and also served as an advertising platform for Vacherie's surgical expertise, however, his own financial motivation was only thinly veiled by such comments.

Vacherie does not hide his excitement about viewing Drouart, despite his ambivalence. Other authors, however, deemphasize their agency and thereby their role in the market for entertainment science. Gottfried Friedrich Burghart, the first German-language author to publish on Drouart, emphasizes that he was not the one who visited Drouart but that, instead, Drouart sought him out: "On May 14 of this year 1763 a Frenchman showed up who requested to talk to me" ["Es war am 14ten Mai dieses 1763 Jahres, als sich bei mir ein Franzos meldete, der mich zu sprechen verlangte"] (15). In line with his critical stance toward developments in the medical profession, Burghart comments on the fact that Drouart "exhibited himself as a natural wonder for money and consequently earned his bread without working" ["sich als Naturwunder vor Geld sehen lassen, folglich sein Brot ohne Arbeiten erwarb"] (19). Burghart demeans Drouart, presenting him either as unwilling to work or as a suspicious salesperson: "What peddler will not praise his goods as much as possible?" ["Und welcher Krämer wird nicht seiner Ware aufs beste loben?"] (21). He never reflects on the circumstances that forced Drouart to exhibit their physique. Burghart highlights the financial incentive for Drouart but never mentions his own as the author of a publication that profits financially and professionally from a disenfranchised individual's predicament.

Unlike Burghart, Heinrich Friederich Delius does not question Drouart's motives. Yet Delius similarly minimizes his own complicity by establishing Drouart as the one who established the encounter. In Delius's description, Drouart seemingly appears out of nowhere, interrupting Delius's anatomical lecture:

> It was this past Winter when, because of a vacant professorship in anatomy, I held splanchnological demonstrations on a female body at the local anatomical theater. While I was busy preparing the inner female reproductive organs the earlier mentioned Drouart appeared, in male clothing, and offered to show himself before the assembled audience.

> I agreed and, after first examining him, showed the pertinent parts at the end of the lecture.
>
> [Es war im verwichenen Winter, als ich wegen damahliger Vacanz der anatomischen Profession an einem weiblichen Körper auf dem hiesigen Theather splanchnologische Demonstrationen hielte. Als ich aber mit der Zubereitung der weiblichen innern Geburts Theile beschäftiget war, meldete sich der erwehnte Drouart, in männlicher Kleidung, bei mir, und erbot sich, vor einer zahlreichen Versammlung sich sehen zu lassen. Ich war wohl damit zufrieden, und nachdem ich ihn zuvor untersuchte, zeigte ich, zu Ende der Vorlesung, and demselben das gehörige.] (399–400)

Delius claims that Drouart themselves offered their body for examination, instead of Delius inviting them to do so. Rather than interrupting his lecture on the body's internal organs, Delius claims that he waited to show Drouart to his students and did so only after having examined him beforehand. In Delius's account, Drouart's appearance at his footstep coincides serendipitously with his demonstration of female reproductive organs. The truth value of this description cannot be ascertained. What is clear, however, is that Delius strives to minimize his own involvement by claiming reticence about exhibiting Drouart's body and raising suspicion about Drouart's trustworthiness.

Debate and Competition

The eighteenth-century creation of the "hermaphrodite" is deeply embedded in physicians' competition in a lucrative marketplace. They felt compelled to comment on famous "hermaphrodites" to prove their relevance. This meant that they had to enter into dialogue with their contemporaries, which could be beneficial as well as detrimental to their professional aspirations. After briefly mentioning the painting by Gautier d'Agoty and the description by Mertrud, Delius references Burghart's "printed news" ["gedruckte Nachricht"] (399), "in which he is inclined to call our Michael Drouart, whom he mistakenly spells Drouet, Maid Anne" ["in welcher er sehr geneigt ist, unsern Michael Drouart, der unrecht Drouet geschrieben ist, für ein Jungfer Annchen zu halten"] (399). Delius directly opposes Burghart's conclusion when he argues that Drouart is a "misshapen man" ["verstaltete Manns-Person"] (404) rather than a woman.

Delius and Burghart were from two different German territories, Nürnberg and Silesia, respectively. Delius's questioning of Burghart's professional judgment therefore had little direct effect either on Delius's or on Burghart's career. In other cases, however, physicians who published on the same case worked in close institutional and regional proximity. On the one hand, voicing a diverging opinion served to assert their professional expertise and superiority. On the other, however, this same move could hurt their career. They therefore had to strategically navigate their professional networks. The case of Maria Dorothea Derrier, who became a patient at the Charité hospital in Berlin, vividly illustrates the careful ways in which medical men positioned themselves. Christoph Wilhelm Hufeland, the Charité's director, published a report on Derrier in 1801; briefly, thereafter, the Charité's chief surgeon, Christian Ludwig Mursinna, published his own study, agreeing with Hufeland's conclusion that Derrier was a woman. Even Monorchis, who satirizes his colleagues' intense focus on "hermaphrodites," does not question Hufeland's assessment.

When Derrier's fame spread beyond Berlin, however, opposing views emerged. Christian Stark, an eminent physician and dean of the medical college in another German intellectual capital—Jena—personally viewed Derrier and used his own journal to contradict Hufeland and Mursinna. In contrast to them, Stark argues that Derrier is a man. He emphasizes that "meticulous researchers" ["genaue Forscher"] (540) have the duty to "examine everything in detail" ["alles genau zu untersuchen"] (540). Describing his own detailed examination thereby casts doubt on those that had taken place previously, namely those by Hufeland and Mursinna. Another physician, Franz Heinrich Martens, further questioned these two medical authorities with his 1802 *Beschreibung und Abbildung einer sonderbaren Misstaltung der männlichen Geschlechtstheile von Maria Dorothea Derrier aus Berlin nebst den Meinungen von Stark, Hufeland, Mursinna und Monorchis über diese Person* [Description and illustration of a peculiar malformation of the male genitals of Maria Dorothea Derrier from Berlin, alongside the opinions of Stark, Hufeland, Mursinna, and Monorchis about this individual]. Martens's study is an independent publication and, at twenty pages, it is the longest on Derrier; it also contains two copperplates, which he claims to be more detailed than previous illustrations. In contrast to the self-confident tone of Stark, dean of the medical college at Jena, anxiety permeates Martens's study. On the one hand, responding to two authorities such as Hufeland and Mursinna serves as a way to assert himself in the medical sphere. On the other, however, this move could be detrimental to his career. Martens therefore strategically flatters Hufeland and Mursinna as "two famous men" ["zwe[i] berühmt[e] Männer"] (5) before proceeding to express doubt about their empirical skills:

> One cannot understand how healthy eyes could have seen such a thing, and the stories in Hufeland's and Mursinna's descriptions are so different from nature itself, from the description by the privy councilor Stark, and from the story repeatedly told to me by the subject itself in Leipzig, that I cannot make sense of them and that I, in order not to offend the literary conscientiousness that both men have as authors, have to conclude that the statements made by the subject in Berlin must have been completely different from those made here and later on in Jena.
>
> [so, daß man nicht begreifen kann, wie man mit gesunden Augen so etwas sehen kann, und die Geschichtserzählungen sind in den Beschreibungen von Hufeland und Mursinna so verschieden von der Natur selbst, von der

> Beschreibung, welche der Hofrath Stark geliefert hat, und von dem, was das Subject mir hier in Leipzig zu wiederholten Malen gleichlautend versicherte, daß ich es schlechterdings nicht zusammen reimen kann, und daß ich, um nicht der schriftstellerischen Gewissenhaftigkeit jener beiden Männer zu nahe zu treten, glauben muß, daß die Aussage der Person selbst in Berlin ganz anders gewesen sei, als sie hier und weiterhin in Jena war.] (5–6)

At the same time that Stark acknowledges Hufeland's and Mursinna's prominence, his questioning of their eyesight functions as an attack on their empirical skills (5). His use of the word "schrifstellerisch" —literary—to refer to their case histories casts doubt on their truthfulness as it suggests that their writing has a literary dimension and might therefore be fictional. His use of the word "reimen" —rhyming—to describe the process by which he tries to make sense of their case histories has similar implications. Stark weakens his criticism of his prominent colleagues by calling into question Derrier's credibility, whom he suspects of having made diverging statements in Berlin and Jena.

Aware of the potential danger of opposing such prominent medical men, Martens explicitly addresses the power dynamics in the eighteenth-century medical sphere: "I would however not have dared publicly to oppose privy councilor Hufeland and general and army surgeon Mursinna, if councilor Stark had not already paved the way" ["Ich hätte es jedoch nicht gewagt, den beiden Schriftstellern, Herrn Geheimen Rath Hufeland, und Herrn General-Staabschirurgus Mursinna öffentlich zu widersprechen, wenn nicht schon der Hofrath Stark die Bahn gebrochen"] (12). Aligning himself with Stark provides Martens with a protective cover. In fact, he agrees with Stark to such an extent "that I have little or nothing to add" ["daß ich wenig oder gar nichts zu derselben hinzuzufügen haben werde"] (13) and concludes that Derrier is "a misshapen man" ["eine misgestaltete Mannsperson"] (17). As a "composite of various opinions" ["Zusammenstellung der verschiedenen Meinungen"]

(6), Martens's *Beschreibung* therefore functions as a reader's digest of all published material on Derrier. Like Parsons before him, Martens not only summarizes previous authors' opinions but also quotes and excerpts from their texts extensively, thereby strategically positioning his text in the market for entertainment science. In contrast to Parsons, however, he references his contemporaries rather than authors from the past. Martens's stated goal is that readers "are no longer misled" ["[sich] … nicht länger … irre führen … lassen"] (20), which allows for his alignment with Stark, who eventually promoted him to a professorial position in his hospital in Jena (Winckel 460–1).

Addenda—Other Cases

Martens's study demonstrates authors' careful negotiation of the publishing realm and their professional networks. In the competitive environment of the eighteenth century, authors not only entered into dialogue with one another regarding the same "hermaphrodite" but also tried to surpass each other by locating other cases of "hermaphroditism" that would prove their theory. At the end of his case history on Drouart, Vacherie mentions that, in Lyon, "there exists actually an Hermaphrodite truly perfect in both Sexes, but that by the Care of the Parents, who are wealthy Merchants, and who will not permit an authentic verification therefore" (14) the matter must remain undecided. This comment highlights the crucial role played by social class in the construction of the category of the "hermaphrodite." After this reference, Vacherie includes a section called "addenda" in which he responds to his critics, who believe that there are no human "hermaphrodites," with a comparative discussion of Drouart and "a Negro Hermophradite [*sic*] from Guinea" (15). In addition to defending his own position, Vacherie's description of this individual allows him to further appeal to his audience's voyeurism. He also establishes a link to Parsons's publication on another African subject, the Angolan "hermaphrodite," which further consolidates the role played by non-European individuals as medical research subjects in the eighteenth century. Similarly, Hoin, at the end of his treatise, included the promise of another case history, "a child born in the vicinity of Dijon" ["un enfant né aux environs de Dijon"] (8). He withholds conclusions, waiting for future developments: "Let us be careful not to predict his future appearance; let us wait at least until puberty" ["Gardons-nous bien de prononcer sur son état futur: attendons qu'il soit parvenu au moins à l'âge de puberté"] (8). By promising a type of sequel, these authors kept their readers engaged and on the lookout for further publications in the same way that writers of serialized fiction did in the eighteenth century.

Other authors such as M. Maret, a surgeon like Vacherie, used the famous Drouart case as a springboard for publishing a study on another "hermaphrodite" who "deserves this name more than all those that Mr. Morand, Metrud, Hoin and Gauthier have had the chance to describe" ["mérite mieux ce nom que tous ceux que Mrs. Morand, Mertrud, Hoin & Gauthier ont eu occasion de décrire"] (157). Maret discusses the case of Hubert-Jean Pierre, a shoemaker apprentice, who develops a fever while living at the master's house. After Pierre dies in the hospital, a nun alerts Maret to the corpse's unusual physique: "The nun who had taken care of him during his illness noticed, when she put a shirt on him, that his breasts were of a size that was not typical for individuals from the male species: this made her doubt his sex" ["La religieuse qui l'avoit servi pendant sa maladie, s'étoit aperçue, en lui passant une chemise, que ce malade avoit des mamelles d'un volume qui n'étoit pas ordinaire aux individus de l'espèce masculine: cela lui inspira des doutes sur son sexe"] (158). The erotic innuendos that permeate this scene position Maret's case history amid similar ones published by his colleagues, among them Hoin. While Maret explicitly challenges Hoin in the introduction, he also invites him to examine the corpse of this "phénomèn[e] extraordinaire[e]" (169). This invitation attests to the close professional medical networks that shaped the scientific book market in the eighteenth century and aligned it with erotic literature of the time. This literature was, like Sade's *Justine*, often set in convents or monasteries and critiqued the ideological underpinnings of the ancien régime.[13] The boudoir and the examination room were the spaces in which eighteenth-century political and scientific change was enacted.

"Hermaphrodite" case histories questioned Enlightenment claims to objectivity and definitive conclusions. Physicians sought to set their inquiries apart from fictional accounts, both past and present, yet the boundaries between science and fiction remained fluid. Because of the open-endedness of case histories, which—like other Enlightenment genres such as the *Encyclopédie*—always gestured toward further updates and revelations, case histories drew on narrative conventions from belles lettres: "Disciplinary boundaries were drawn in the name of objectivity, to excise messy cultural attitudes from the scientific enterprise, but the storytelling mode of case histories consistently undermines their supposed objectivity" (Tougaw 4). The genre of the case history sought to consolidate the separation between scientific and literary writing, yet through its narrativity, questioned this dichotomy. In fact, the "hermaphrodite" as a category of medical and popular curiosity came into being at the intersection of these two genres, which were imbued with "uncertainities that fueled narrative desire" (10). The narrative creation of the "hermaphrodite" in eighteenth-century discourse curtailed any direct reflection on the ethical issues posed by the disadvantaged status of the individuals in question. As Chapter 3 will show, medical discourse's bringing into being of the "hermaphrodite" was closely linked to and shaped by the desire to unlock the broader secrets of human generation and reproduction. Individuals whom the medical establishment considered to resist categorization within the heterosexual model of reproduction were pathologized and dehumanized.

Notes

1 For a discussion of Hufeland and the status of medicine in the eighteenth century, see Pfeifer.

2 An overview of the development of the technical press is provided in Kronick, *A History*.

3 Only wealthy buyers could have afforded the intricate artwork depicting "hermaphrodites" produced by, for example, Moreau le Jeune, or included in the *Encyclopédie*.

4 Dirks-Schuster discusses the multiple connections between print culture and the scientific and popular interest in "hermaphrodites" in the early modern period.

5 In Prussia, Frederick the Great introduced compulsory education in 1763. In other German territories and European countries, this happened much later, in the late nineteenth century in the case of France and Britain. Even in those territories, however, before education became mandatory, there existed schools that were becoming increasingly accessible to children. As R. A. Houston demonstrates, attendance varied greatly and depended not only on social class and gender but also on cultural attitudes toward education (11–60). On the case of Prussia in particular, see Van Horn Melton. For France and Britain and the role of gender in education, see de Bellaigue.

6 For changes in the eighteenth-century book market, among others, see Runge and Rogers, Raven, Rivers (English); Bohm, Jefcoate, Bell (German); and Mark Curran, Darnton (French).

7 Ian Watt's 1957 *The Rise of the Novel* significantly shaped literary history's interpretation of the rise of fiction. In the more than six decades since Watt, scholars have complicated his thesis, addressing Watt's exclusion of women authors and his description of the genre's emergence in ex nihilo fashion. For a discussion of responses to Watt, see Hilger, *Women* 11–20. One of the most recent critiques of Watt's thesis can be found in Frank.

8 In addition to Robert Darnton's groundbreaking work on eighteenth-century publishing, a discussion of the intersection between pornography and the novel can be found in Marcus and Toulalan, *Imagining Sex*, for the British context; DeJean (all), Goulemot, and Jacob for France; and Sangmeister and Mulsow for German-speaking lands.

9 On the blurring of the line between scientific writing and erotica/pornography during this period, also see Harvey, Traub.

10 Since the textual elements of eighteenth-century medical case histories on "hermaphrodites" have traditionally not been read against the grain, this book quotes passages at length and unpacks them in detail. By contrast, the illustrations

included in these case histories have been reproduced and analyzed in depth in previous publications such as those by Graille, Schochow, and Courtney Thompson. I have therefore decided not to include visual representations, in order to lessen the potentially triggering effect of analyzing these medical case histories.

11 See Gayatri Chakravorty Spivak's essay "Can the Subaltern Speak?" for a discussion of the concept of subalternity in the postcolonial context.

12 See Marguillier for information about Simon's life and work.

13 DeJean's "The Politics" discusses pornography's political critique in the eighteenth century.

3

Reproduction: Fluids and Other Matters

Physicians and surgeons constructed the "hermaphrodite" by observing, measuring, and describing individuals with variable sex characteristics. Despite their seemingly decisive pronouncements, which either strategically aligned with or contradicted their predecessors, ambiguity permeated their writing. Jacques Louis Hoin, for example, concluded that "he [Michel-Anne Drouart] hoped to become a mother" ["il espéroit devenir mère"] (7). Hoin strongly argued for Drouart being reassigned as female yet he used the male pronoun, which undermined his seeming certainty, thereby creating a space for nonbinary sex, the existence of which he explicitly denied. In addition to revealing Hoin's ambivalence, the use of the male pronoun in conjunction with a reference to female generation points to the centrality of the issue of reproduction in debates concerning individuals with nonstandard sexual anatomy. As Jason Farr has argued, "Impaired bodies are … fundamental to the cultural construction of homo- and heterosexuality" (2). The attempt to classify "hermaphroditic" bodies as either male or female "expose[s] able-bodiedness and heterosexuality as imbricated systems that sustain dominant models of reproductive futurity" (1). The eighteenth-century construction of the "hermaphrodite" as an object of study was therefore not merely auxiliary but central to discussions about the process by which normative bodies reproduced.

In their attempt to answer questions about "hermaphrodites'" reproductive potential, medical practitioners provided detailed descriptions of their visible genitals and their functioning. These accounts aligned with the empirical drive that was connected to the changes in the medical realm and the popularization of scientific literature. Medical case histories investigated and described a living and breathing subject. In contrast to autopsy reports, which were mainly of interest to medical specialists, case histories appealed to a much broader audience. These studies functioned similarly to the popular novels of the time, focusing on the adversities faced by the protagonist. Readers' curiosity about a specific "hermaphrodite's" fate triggered the production of "sequels" by scientists throughout Europe; this sequelization was both a cause for and a result of the reading public's voyeuristic interest in stories with erotic and even pornographic content as well as a growing interest in natural history. At the same time that examining a living body limited physicians to the external genitals, it also allowed them to record the "hermaphrodite's" reactions to their probing and prodding. The relationship between scientist and "hermaphrodite" mirrors that between aristocratic rogue and bourgeois virgin in eighteenth-century novels. The power differential and violence were central to the heteronormative plot that often culminated in offspring or the future promise thereof.

In medical case histories, authors rarely reflect explicitly on the ethics of their painfully graphic descriptions that are framed with the language of empirical science. This absence only heightens the question of the audience's implication in the construction of these bodies in the medical and the popular imagination. In this respect, medical case histories pose the question of moral sensibility that Kathleen Lubey discusses in the context of erotic fiction, which invites readers to stop and think about their own moral character in the middle of detailed descriptions of physical encounters. The tension between readers' desire for salacious details and the discomfort in witnessing scenes of violence and rape creates an unsettling complicity. This complicity needs to be acknowledged before closely reading narratives about these nonbinary individuals in order to expose and thereby denaturalize their construction of "hermaphrodites" and related notions of reproduction.

Clitoris and Penis—Ovaries and Testicles

In their studies, scientists established a map of the "hermaphrodite's" body at the center of which stood the external genitals as privileged signifiers. The penis played a predominant role, and scientists strove to distinguish it from the clitoris. The attempt to demarcate male from female organs questioned theories about sexual difference that had been popular since Galenic times. For Galen (129–210 CE), who based his thinking on Hippocratic humoral medicine, men and women consisted of the same basic structures. The main difference was that women were seen as inferior versions of the male ideal. The clitoris was, for example, a smaller version of the penis. Similarly, the ovaries were considered to be the female counterpart of the testicles, only hidden inside the woman's abdominal cavity. The fact that ovaries and testicles had both been called stones for centuries—preceded by either the modifier "male" or "female"—testifies to this homologic thinking. Humoral medicine posited that women produced less body heat than men and therefore burned off less excess blood through sweat (Lisa Smith, "The Body" 26–46).[1] As a result of this supposed deficiency, women's bodies resorted to compensatory mechanisms such as menstruation to maintain and reestablish the balance of the four humors: blood, phlegm, black bile, and yellow bile. Eighteenth-century anatomists gradually began to think outside the explanatory framework of the one-sex model, in which women were similar, yet lesser versions, of men. Instead, they began to consider the sexes as incommensurably different, as Thomas Laqueur has put it. This shift from the one- to the two-sex model most visibly affected the conceptualization of the genitals. Describing Michel-Anne Drouart's physique, Heinrich Friederich Delius observes "quite a respectable male member with glans and foreskin" ["ein ganz ansehnliches männliches Glied mit seiner Eichel und Vorhaut"] (401) and insists that it "did not have any resemblance at all with an elongated clitoris" ["hatte ganz und gar keine Aehnlichkeit mit einer verlängerten Clitoris"] (401). Similarly, Burghart describes "a member … without which no one can be called a man" ["ein Glied … ohne welches niemand ein Mannsperson heissen kan"] (17). However, despite the similarity in their observations, these two men come to opposite conclusions. Whereas Delius decides that the presence of a sizable penis signifies Drouart's masculinity, for Burghart, this structure is an "unnatural growth" ["widernatürliche[s] Gewächse"] (18) that should be surgically removed to allow Drouart to continue life as a woman.

For every scientist who strove to establish penis and clitoris as opposite structures, however, another one argued that these two structures shared the same anatomy. This lack of consensus shows that the shift from the one- to the two-sex model of sex and gender was a gradual and contested process. In this respect, Antoine Ferrein's conclusion to his *Mémoire sur le véritable sexe* (1767) demonstrates the persistence of the one-sex model in the eighteenth century particularly forcefully: "Even the lesser anatomists know that the clitoris or the female member only differs from that of the male in its small size and the lack of a urethra and that, otherwise, it is formed the same as that of men" ["Les moindres Anatomistes savent que le clitoris ou la verge féminine, ne diffère guère de celle de l'homme que par la petitesse & par le défaut de l'urètre, qu'elle est formée d'ailleurs comme chez les hommes"] (336).

In their search for answers, physicians not only described the genitals' appearance but also strove to elucidate their functioning in a living individual. These descriptions are extremely detailed and graphic, projecting readers into an uncomfortable voyeuristic position as they are reading about aspects of real individuals' bodies and lives that are typically kept private. Describing

Drouart, Sauveur-François Morand relates both what he himself observed and what the "hermaphrodite" reported: Drouart "often experiences, upon waking, an erection of varying strength, which lasts for about an hour … he does not care to provoke it outside of these circumstances and says that it is very difficult for him, albeit possible" ["a souvent à son réveil, de l'érection plus ou moins forte, qui se soutient environ une heure de suite … il ne se soucie point de se la provoquer hors de ces deux circonstances, & dit que cela lui est fort difficile, quoique possible"] ("Description" 3–4). Morand uses Drouart's reported erections as proof of masculinity. Franz Heinrich Martens follows a similar line of reasoning when he claims that Derrier's "male member" ["männliches Glied"] "could easily be brought into a state of erection through friction" ["ließ sich durch Friktion leicht in Erektion bringen"] (15). Christian Ludwig Mursinna also reports that an erection was discovered on Derrier's body by "surgeons in the Charité, in the morning during sleep" ["Chirurgen in der Charitée, des Morgens im Schlaf"] (557). Unlike Martens, however, Mursinna does not use erections as proof of Derrier's masculinity, pointing instead at their ambiguous meaning. At the same time that these physicians strove to differentiate penis and clitoris, the homology of the one-sex model persisted. The fact that Martens uses the phrase "ein männliches Glied," a male penis/member, implies the possibility of a female penis/member. In fact, Ferrein's reference to a "verge féminine" ["female penis"] further cements the analogy between penile and clitoral structures. The excerpts from these case histories show that the line between male and female genitals remained blurry regardless of forceful attempts to fixate it. As Ula Lukszo Klein observes, despite the aggressive defense and reification of the gender binary in the eighteenth century, a close reading of texts produced during this time period uncovers the "inherent nonbinarism of gender" (12). As a result, "the penis is and is not a marker of maleness in these texts" (26). The "hermaphrodite's" body frustrates the scientist's goal of establishing clear classifications, prompting him to perform increasingly invasive physical exams.

Semen

As the anatomy and functioning of the genitals did not fully answer physicians' questions, they turned to genital secretions. Jean Jacques Louis Hoin, who believed that female characteristics dominated in Drouart, describes the results of Drouart's daydreaming as "a half-voluptuous awakening that caused the natural excretion of a limpid humor in his/her[2] vagina" ["un réveil à demi voluptueux, en occasionnant dans son vagin l'excrétion naturelle d'une humeur limpide"] (7). Morand similarly states that Drouart claimed that "at the end of the erection he feels an intense and pleasurable tickling sensation on the inside and that, in those moments, it seems that something warm escapes but he does not know in what area" ["il dit qu'à la fin de l'érection il sent au dedans un chatouillement très-vif qui lui fait plaisir, & que dans ce temps-là il lui semble que quelque chose de chaud s'échappe, sans qu'il sache dans quelle partie"] ("Description" 4). Lost in the internal recesses of Drouart's enigmatic genitals, this fluid does not provide any answers. The fact that Hoin calls the emitted bodily fluid a "limpid humor" and that Vacherie describes Drouart's emissions as "certain humours or Seminal Fluids" (12) testifies to the persistence of Galenic humoral thinking and the porous borders between the sexes, despite all assertions to the contrary. While new theories about reproduction, most prominently preformation and epigenesis—which will be discussed later in this chapter—percolated throughout the eighteenth century, Galen's notion that both men and women experienced erections and produced semen, with the female one being weaker and colder, persisted both in medical literature and the popular imagination (Wiesner-Hanks, *Women* 31).[3]

By the mid-eighteenth century, the description of seminal fluids had become a convention of the "hermaphrodite" case history genre and its absence was noted, similarly to that of accompanying illustrations. In his 1768 *Dissertation sur les hermaphrodites*, a review of the most famous case histories, Arnaud

Ronsil laments the lack of any description by Vermeil and Champeaux of "the nature of the liquid that Grandjean produced in all likelihood" ["la nature de la liqueur que Grandjean devoit vraisemblablement produire"] (388). In the eighteenth century, these bodily liquids were seen as central not only to the scientific quest to discover the "hermaphrodite's" "true" sex but also to the voyeurism that propelled the marketing of these case histories. Despite the focus on these emissions, however, none of the case histories reference a microscopic examination of them. Considering the discovery of moving organisms in seminal fluid by Antonie van Leeuwenhoek in the late seventeenth century, this absence is telling in a period that foregrounded empiricism above all.[4] The meaning of Leeuwenhoek's discovery of these "animalcules"—which we now know to be spermatozoa—was far from clear when it occurred and remained so throughout the eighteenth century. Various theories regarding the animalcules were proposed, ranging from a fertilizing agent to an entity that kept sperm from coagulating (Pranghofer 174–5 and Toulalan, "Unfit" 304). Because seminal fluid remained an ambiguous signifier, its microscopic examination would not have yielded the type of definitive results that scientists were pursuing. Moreover, the results of such investigations would not have fit the genre of the "hermaphrodite" case histories, which was also geared at a broad audience interested in (salacious) details regarding the lives and loves of ambiguously sexed humans and not only at medical specialists curious about the results of microscopic exams of genital emissions.

Menstrual Blood

Because of the ambivalent nature of the newly discovered "animalcules" in semen, the line between semen and other bodily emissions, in particular menstrual blood, remained fluid, as it had been since Galenic times. Semen was considered to be made from blood and in "a complicated process of concoction it became 'a frothy Liquor'" (Toulalan, "Unfit" 307). In a similarly complex operation, menstrual blood—which was thought to emanate from the gallbladder to nourish the fetus during pregnancy—was transformed into breast milk (Read 11).[5] Blood was blood but it could also be transformed into another liquid. Therefore, rather than being completely different, blood and semen were considered to be related emissions, which made it difficult to invoke them as determining factors for determining "hermaphrodites'" "true" sex. Like semen, menstrual blood was an ambivalent signifier in more than one way. Menstrual blood was less likely to be spotted during an examination and, unlike semen, could not be provoked, either by the "hermaphrodite" or the physician. Therefore, scientists' only source of information was the "hermaphrodite's" own account. Morand and Vacherie, examining Drouart at the age of sixteen, claim the absence of menstrual flow yet leave room for the possibility that it might appear in the future because of "certain Symptoms, however equivocal, there is some room to conjecture, that it will not even want that Sign of the Female Sex" (Vacherie 13). Examining Drouart more than a decade later, Burghart, Delius, Ferrein, and Hoin report, "The correct tribute every month, even though not in abundance" ["richtig alle Monat den gewöhnlichen Tribut, ob zwar nicht in allzu reichlicher Menge"] (Burghart 19), "some blood" ["etwas Geblüt"] (Delius 402), and "her period, even though it was not abundant" ["ses règles, sans être abondantes"] (Ferrein 338). Hoin states that Drouart's "period … began to emerge … between her twentieth and twenty-first year … it occurs exactly every month" ["règles … ont commence à paroître … entre l'âge de vingt & vingt-un ans … elles ont leur cours exactement tous les mois"] (6). Despite physicians' search for menstrual blood, however, its presence did not mean that Drouart was unequivocally a woman.

The authors all emphasize that the information regarding menstrual flow was obtained not through their own firsthand observation but that it was reported by Drouart. Their goal in mentioning this, however, varies and depends on whether they categorize Drouart as male or female. Burghart, making the case that Drouart should live life as a woman, mentions that Drouart "repeatedly affirmed" ["unter wiederholtem Bejahen"] (19) that they menstruated. Hoin, in agreement with Burghart, argues that a firsthand witnessing of Drouart's period—"this critical state" ["cet état critique"]—was "at present not necessary to characterize her dominant sex" ["à present peu nécessaire pour caractériser son sexe dominant"] (6) because of an abundance of other female anatomical indicators. Delius, by contrast, casts doubt on Drouart's description: "Out of the same vagina flowed urine and, as Drouart wanted to assure me, some blood at certain times. But I did not see it and he only said that it was not that time. He probably said the same thing in all other places" ["Aus derselben [Scheide] gieng der Urin, und, wie Drouart versichern wollte, zu gewissen Zeiten etwas Geblüt. Ich habe es aber nicht gesehen, und er sagte nur, daß es eben die periodische Zeit nicht wäre. So hat er aber vermuthlich an allen Orten auch gesagt"] (402). Delius, who categorized Drouart as male, questions the veracity of the "hermaphrodite's" statements. He also suggests that Drouart is parroting other medical men when he comments that Drouart called their own external genitals "the vagina, because that is what he had been told" ["la vagine, die Scheide, weil man es ihm ohnehin so vorgesagt"] (402). Delius's patronizing approach here mirrors his questioning of Drouart's motives for exhibiting their body, which he interprets as a lack of the desire to work. At the same time, however, the reader gets glimpses of the "hermaphrodite's" subjectivity. Albeit mediated by the physician, Drouart's awareness and understanding of medical discourse emerges in this excerpt.

Whereas most authors discussing Drouart devote a phrase, a line, or at most a paragraph to the question of menstruation, Ferrein spends two entire pages exploring it. In contrast to Delius, Ferrein underlines Drouart's trustworthiness. He strategically claims that Drouart is not familiar with medical discourse when he argues that those are "circumstances that someone who, like him, does not know medicine could never invent" ["circonstances qu'un ignorant en Médicine, tel que lui, ne sauroit jamais inventer"] (337). He also posits that there are no contradictions in Drouart's account—"without contradicting himself on anything at all" ["sans se contredire sur quoi que ce soit"] (337). Rather than questioning Drouart's credibility, Ferrein emphasizes the "hermaphrodite's" own empirical skills, which align with the physician's examinations, which Ferrein performed twice, three months apart. According to Ferrein, Drouart's menstrual secretions appeared at the age of seventeen as "a viscous and yellowish liquor, the quantity of which could reach half a cup in twenty-four hours" ["une liqueur visqueuse & jaunâtre, dont la quantité pouvoit aller à un demi-goblet en vingt-quatre heures"] (337). The liquid's consistency and color resemble semen more than blood; it thereby further blurs the line between male and female genital emissions. While this "liquour" itself does not appear exclusively menstrual, the accompanying symptoms do: "He had strong headaches and colics, his bosom swelled, the top of the nipples became painful and his attempts to touch them produced shooting pains" ["il eut des grands maux de tête & des coliques, le sein se gonfla, le bout des mamelles devint douloureux avec des élancements lorsqu'il vouloit y toucher"] (337–8). Drouart explained to Ferrein that this liquid appeared for four years and then "his period became completely irregular and even ceased after a certain time" ["ses règles se dérangèrent totalement & cessèrent même au bout de quelque temps"] (338). However, Ferrein also reports Drouart's assertion that "since then, he has sometimes seen some red, but rarely and very little … nothing has appeared for eight months" ["depuis cela, il a vu quelquefois en rouge, mais rarement & fort peu … il y avoit huit mois que rien n'avoit paru"] (338). The period-like emissions seem to have ceased but Ferrein suggests that they might reappear at any time.

For Ferrein, the disappearance of menstrual discharge does not mean that Drouart is not a woman. Even though he uses a male pronoun, he considers Drouart a woman. Ferrein echoes humoral theories on menstruation when he argues that "this is probably the result of the significant movement and the continuous travelling in which he has engaged for so many years" ["c'est sans doute l'effet des grands exercices & voyages continuels qu'il a faits depuis tant d'années"] (338). Menstruation was seen as a biological necessity to burn off excess blood due to women's supposedly colder nature and their sedentary life style. Therefore, if women increased their physical activity, Ferrein conjectures, regular and copious menstruation was no longer necessary to maintain humoral balance.

In the Grandjean case, the lawyer Champeaux similarly explores the ambiguity of menstrual flow to argue that Grandjean should continue life as a woman, invoking the authority of the Greek physician Galen: "Women who work in tiring professions only have very light flow and the most robust ones are the ones who typically have none, as Galen has observed" ["Les femmes occupées à des travaux fatiguants n'ont que de très légers écoulements; & les plus robustes en sont les plus exemptes, comme l'a observé Galien"] (Champeaux 52–3). Champeaux comments on the absence of menstruation in Grandjean, ascribing it to physical exertion, even though Françoise Lambert, Grandjean's companion, "assured me that Grandjean was subject to this evacuation" ["assure que la Grand-Jean est sujette à cette evacuation"] (52). This poses two questions: first, whether Champeaux doubted Lambert's trustworthiness, and second, whether Lambert ever wondered about her husband's menstruation if it did, indeed, occur. The answer to these questions might not matter in retracing the construction of Grandjean as a "hermaphrodite" since genital bleeding continued to have more than one meaning in the eighteenth century. Despite Grandjean's menstruation, Lambert never questioned her spouse's masculinity, as reported by Vermeil: "Ils vivoient dans la bonne foi heureux & tranquilles, sans que Françoise Lambert eût aucune défiance du sexe de son mari, & sans que ce mari eût aucun soupçon de son insuffisance" ["They lived happily and quietly in good faith, without Françoise Lambert having any distrust about her husband's sex, & without this husband having any suspicion of his insufficiency"] (5–6). Vermeil's focus on the heterosexual nature of their relationship cements his claim that Grandjean should continue to live as a man, whereas Champeaux' reflections on menstrual fluid align with his conclusion that Grandjean is a woman. In either case history, menstruation functioned as an ambivalent signifier.

Male Menstruation

The absence or presence of menstrual flow did not necessarily qualify or disqualify an individual for or from womanhood. Conversely, because periodic bloody emissions were not seen as an absolute marker of femininity, their presence did not necessarily mean that the individual could not be a man. Grandjean's case illustrates this particularly forcefully; Grandjean's wife never thought that her husband was not a man, despite episodes of genital bleeding. In this context, Cathy McClive argues that, in the eighteenth century, "male periodic bleeding [was located] within humoral notions of healthy balance" (206).[6] Like women, male bodies could suffer from an excess of blood, leading to "nosebleeds, coughing up blood, or bleeding haemorrhoids" (Lisa Smith, "An Unusual" 5). Similarly, Gianna Pomata posits that periodic bleeding in men—male menstruation—was considered healthy and was associated with longevity and fertility. The first-century author Plinius was still quoted on this point in the eighteenth century and rhythmical change remained a cornerstone in the understanding of the human body (Stolberg, "Menstruation" 97). From this perspective, the female body provided a model through which to understand its male counterpart; this interpretive framework turned on its head the notion that the male was the more perfect one in the one-sex model.[7] The common eighteenth-century practice of bloodletting to cure a variety of ailments fits this understanding of the human body.[8]

Discussions of Derrier's case engage the notion of male periodic bleeding. While Hufeland and Mursinna use the presence of menstrual fluid, however irregular, as proof of Derrier's womanhood, for Stark the meaning of this bleeding is less clear: "That, once, and only this one time, after a fall and an illness, she had seen some blood emanate from the orifice, but this also often happens to men in other instances, from the urethra" ["daß sie zwar einmal, aber nur ein einzigesmal nach einem Fall und einer Krankheit etwas Blutiges aus der Oeffnung kommen gesehen, welches aber auch oft bei Mannspersonen in andern Fällen zuweilen aus der Harnröhre erfolgt"] (in Martens 17, Stark 646). Stark argues that "one should definitely not conclude from this event the presence of monthly flow" ["daraus darf man durchaus nicht auf das Daseyn des Monatlichen schließen"] (in Martens 17, Stark 646). Stark's dismissal of Derrier's bleeding as the result of disease or injury aligns with his assessment of Derrier as a man. It does not, however, completely eliminate the possibility of male periodic bleeding. Even though Stark claims that Derrier only experienced this type of bleeding once—"ein einzigesmal"—he mentions two instances, a fall and an illness, before obliquely referring to other examples. Stark classifies Derrier more ambiguously than he wants to, as can be seen in his pronouncement that Derrier is a man while using the female pronoun "sie."

The notion of male periodic bleeding, itself predicated on female menstruation, opened the possibility of female periodic bleeding through other body parts, such as the nose, the lungs, and the bowels. At a time when menstrual blood was thought to emanate from the gallbladder, an organ common to both sexes, "leaky male bodies" (Lisa Smith, "The Body" 26) complicated the relationship between genital bleeding and biological sex. Because periodic bleeding was not exclusive to women it was not an absolute signifier of womanhood. In this context it bears reminding that, while menstruation was linked to reproduction in the second half of the eighteenth century, the link to ovulation was only made in the 1870s.[9]

Shaping Bodies

The meaning of genital bleeding was particularly ambiguous in the case of "hermaphrodites" who regularly underwent invasive and painful anatomical examinations. Hoin, for example, describes Drouart as being "very sensitive when the probe was introduced; ordinarily some droplets of blood appeared" ["fort sensible au moment de l'introduction de la sonde; elle fait meme ordinairement sortir quelques gouttelettes de sang"] (5). Repeated examinations could cause episodes of bleeding, of variable intensity and at various moments. In fact, as Hoin points out, it was unusual for the "hermaphrodite" not to bleed: "This time, Drouart barely experienced the kind of pain that he typically feels when the probe is inserted and no blood emerged" ["Cette fois, Drouart n'a presque point éprouvé la douleur qu'il a coutume de ressentir quand on le sonde, & il n'est point sorti de sang"] (5). The absence of blood was so unusual that it needed to be mentioned.

Genital bleeding was therefore both a cause and an effect of being a "hermaphrodite" in the eighteenth century. Medical men literally shaped the "hermaphrodite's" body through their examinations, as becomes clear in Mursinna's voyeuristically explicit descriptions of his violent handling of Derrier's body:

> I could not only immediately insert the tip of my small finger more than one inch and see the opening of the urethra in the front and toward the upper part of this opening but was also able, because of this, to insert a female catheter, in addition to my finger, into the bladder and empty the urine. As a result, I managed to insert half of my index finger because the entrance to the vagina had been widened somewhat by several attempts. Because this caused her pain and she quickly recoiled, I was not able to probe any further.
>
> [Ich konnte nicht nur gleich, die Spitze meines kleinen Fingers über einen Zoll tief hineinbringen, auch die Eröffnung der Harnröhre, vorn und etwas nach oben, in dieser Öffnung wahrnehmen, sondern dadurch auch, neben meinem Finger, einen weiblichen Catheder bis in die Blase führen und den Harn ausleeren. In der Folge, da der Eingang in die Scheide, durch mehrere

Versuche etwas mehr erweitert war, vermochte ich auch meinen Zeigefinger über die Hälfte einzuführen. Da dies ihr aber Schmerzen verursachte, und sie sich schnell zurückzog, vermochte ich nicht höher zu dringen] (556–7)

Mursinna describes the gradual process by which he expands Derrier's vagina. Hiding behind medicine's empiricism, he appeals to his reader's voyeurism with this minute description of his detailed exams. He also references several attempts at expanding the entrance to the vagina, which are either his own or those by other physicians. While Mursinna does not mention any bleeding, Derrier's pain suggests its possibility. Mursinna reflects on further widening the vagina: "Even though the vagina was narrow, it was long and expandable … In all likelihood it could be further expanded through repeated attempts and could be made capable for intercourse" ["Die Scheide war zwar enge, aber doch lang, ausdehnungsfähig … Höchstwahrscheinlich würde sie durch wiederholte Bemühungen mehr ausgedehnt, und zum Beischlaf fähig werden] (558). The invasiveness of Mursinna's examination foreshadows the role that surgeons, from the nineteenth century onwards, would play in shaping genitals that were considered nonstandard in order to render heterosexual intercourse possible. Ferrein similarly remarks on the narrowness of Drouart's vagina and compares it to that of a female virgin:

One knows that in girls who have not been deflowered and in particular in those who have not yet reached puberty, the hymen and the four mounds that have been called caroncules myrtiformes by anatomists of the past century, render the entrance to the vagina extremely narrow and that sometimes the hymen does not permit any passage.

[On sait que chez les filles qui n'ont pas été déflorées, & particulièrement chez celles qui n'ont pas attaint l'âge de puberté, l'hymen & les quatre eminences nommées caroncules myrtiformes par les Anatomistes du siècle passé, rendent l'entrée du vagin extrèmement étroite, & et même que l'hymen ne laisse quelquefois aucun passage.] (334)

Male intervention is presented as necessary to transform the ambiguous or immature body into a full-fledged woman. Ferrein's voyeuristic description echoes rape scenes in sentimental and pornographic fiction of the time. The physician in the case history and the aristocratic rogue in eighteenth-century fiction play a similar role in narratives that seek to enforce a heteronormative plot at a time when bodies were, despite all assertions to the contrary, not viewed as static entities.

Ula Lukszo Klein has observed that, in the eighteenth century, bodies were considered malleable and could be shaped, not only by medical men but also by the bearers themselves. Discussing "hermaphrodites" in general, Stark mentions "a woman with a somewhat elongated clitoris, with which she was either born or which she elongated through self-stimulation" ["ein Frauenzimmer mit einem etwas verlängerten Kitzler (clitoris), der ihm entweder angebohren war, oder den es sich durch Selbstreitz verlängert hatte"] (539). Stark's erotic-scientific description suggests that genitals were moldable as a result of active intervention such as masturbation. They could also be hiding inside the body, as Stark conjectures regarding Derrier's testicles. He argues that, while testicles are typically visible, they might be concealed inside the abdomen: "But the area surrounding the right groin … seemed to be swollen and it was very flexible" ["Doch war die rechte Leistengegend … wie geschwollen, auch sehr elastisch"] (645). He "is confident when he conjectures that it was a testicle that was still sitting behind the abdominal ring" ["glaub[t] sicher vermuthen zu dürfen, daß es ein Testikel war, der noch hinter dem Bauchring sass"] (547). Martens similarly suspects a testicle in the abdominal ring and reports Derrier's description of "a dragging pain in the abdominal ring, up towards the hypochondrial region" ["ein empfindliches Ziehen vom Bauchring aufwärts nach den Hypochondrien"] (17) during erections. The meaning of this hidden signifier was ambivalent at a time when the homology of the "stones"—either male or female—persisted in both popular and medical discourse. For Martens, Derrier is a woman, while Stark considers Derrier a man. Not having a visible testicle did not disqualify Derrier from manhood. And, conversely, having a hidden testicle did not mean that Derrier could not be a woman.

Love Interests

Scientists investigated "hermaphrodites'" genitals and their functioning in hopes of determining their reproductive potential. It is no coincidence that Delius calls them the "birthing parts" ["Geburts Theile"] (401). Discussing Derrier, Mursinna wonders "whether she could be impregnated" ["[o]b sie beschwängert werden könnte"] (558). One central element in this inquiry was the attempt to determine an individual's sexual orientation, always in view of establishing the heterosexual conditions that would render reproduction possible. These inquiries not only served a medical purpose but also appealed to readers interested in salacious details of the "hermaphrodite's" life. As was the case with the description of "hermaphrodites'" menstruation, scientists had to rely on their subject's accounts for determining their sexual orientation. This reversed power dynamic points at one of the few moments of agency that "hermaphrodites" had in shaping the medical narrative about them and, to some extent, their assignment as either male or female. Those medical men who concluded that their object of study was a man all mention Derrier's attraction to the female sex. Martens, for example, describes Derrier as having "much inclination towards the female sex" ["viel Neigung zum weiblichen Geschlecht"] (17). Discussing Drouart, Morand observes "a pronounced inclination towards girls" ["une inclination décidée pour les filles"] ("Description" 4) and Delius asserts somewhat more tentatively "that he was not completely indifferent towards women and noticed occasionally that certain stimuli caused the described member to harden and bend ["dass er gegen Frauens Personen nicht ganz gleichgültig seie, und zuweilen auch besondere Reize und eine Steifigkeit und Krümme des gemeldeten Theiles merke"] (404). Morand's conclusion that Drouart is a man is based not only on their attraction toward women but also on their unresponsiveness to the male scientist's probing fingers. The resulting description encapsulates the violence and power dynamic in these medical encounters; Drouart is the subject of scientific rape by the physician: "He is not at all responsive to the introduction of the finger into the female part, not even to the movements made to stimulate it" ["Il n'est point du tout sensible à l'introduction du doigt dans la partie feminine, même aux movemens qu'on ferait pour l'exciter"] ("Description" 4). Conversely, Ferrein uses Drouart's reaction to his examination as proof that Drouart is indeed a woman: "I inserted the small finger … Michel told me that the insertion of the small finger caused a certain tickling sensation, a lascivious impression" ["j'y introduis le petit doigt … Michel me dit que chez lui l'introduction du petit doigt causoit un certain chatouillemnt, une impression lascive"] (335). Having or not having a pleasurable sensation to an invasive physical examination is, paradoxically, interpreted as an indicator of the "hermaphrodite's" sexual orientation. The physician deploys the same violence as the aristocratic rogue in eighteenth-century fiction; both assert their power over the bodies of those who have little control over their own lives.

While Ferrein sees Drouart's supposedly favorable reaction to his prodding fingers as proof of femininity, those scientists who conclude that their subject is a woman typically comment on her passionlessness. Describing Derrier, Hufeland observes that "no trace was found of an active sexual drive; on the contrary, on all occasions there was feminine coyness, virginity, and decency" ["[m]an hat keine Spur eines regen Geschlechtstriebes entdecken können, vielmehr zeigte sich bei allen Gelegenheiten weibliche Verschämtheit,

Jungfräulichkeit und Decenz"] (171). Monorchis similarly comments that "she is not at all inclined towards either sex" ["[v]on einer gewissen Neigung zu dem einen oder anderen Geschlecht will sie durchaus nichts wissen"] (6). Hufeland's and Monorchis's view of women as passionless fits the emerging two-sex model. In the sixteenth and the seventeenth centuries, the importance of female sexual pleasure and orgasm in conception had been emphasized due to the rediscovery of the two-seed theory of Hippocrates and Galen. This theory enabled a more egalitarian model of procreation than the Middle Ages (McLaren 323–41) through a new valuation of the clitoris.[10] By contrast, eighteenth-century scientists shifted to a view of women as comparatively passionless, which made female sexual arousal immaterial for reproduction. Laqueur argues that "female orgasm, which had been the body's signal of successful generation, was banished to the borderlands of physiology, a signifier without a signified" (150). "Orgasm became a player in the game of new sexual differences" (150) where it was constructed as important only for men. The discussion of sexual arousal was therefore central in "hermaphrodite" case histories in the attempt to demarcate clitoris and penis. As scientists sought to differentiate these two structures, however, sexual arousal necessarily remained an ambivalent signifier, which—far from providing conclusive answers—raised even more questions, also with respect to the problematic and violent ways in which physicians sought to elicit it in their objects of study.

Reproducing Bodies

In their attempts to determine the possibility of heterosexual relations and therefore reproduction, medical men not only examined but also proposed to alter the bodies they were examining. Hoin claims that Drouart is "animated by the natural desire to contribute to the propagation of the human species, he hoped to become a mother; we do not see any physical hurdle to him achieving this goal after undergoing the surgery that we suggest" ["animé par le désir naturel de contribuer à la propagation de l'espèce humaine, il espéreroit devenir mere [*sic*]; qualité que nous ne voyons rien qui puisse l'empêcher d'acquérir physiquement, après qu'il auroit souffert l'opération proposée"] (7). Hoin, who uses the male pronoun to refer to Drouart, stipulates that he would perform the operation, which he calls a "debridement of the vagina" ["débridement du vagin"] (7), only if Drouart wants to marry and therefore reproduce (7). Delius, who considers Drouart a "misshapen man" ["verstaltete Manns Person"], does not suggest altering Drouart's body because, according to him, surgery would not change the fact that "he cannot beget" ["er nicht zeugen kann"] (404). Hoin and Delius strive to determine Drouart's reproductive potential as either man or woman. Vacherie, by contrast, is the only proponent of the idea that Drouart, to whom he refers with the pronoun "it," is a "true" "hermaphrodite" who might be capable of the "double Act of Generation" (13). At the same time that this belief in humans with doubled reproductive potential aligns Vacherie with old theories of "hermaphroditism," it also allows him to position his treatise in the new marketplace for entertainment science more forcefully than his colleagues. After all, a true "hermaphrodite" was more intriguing to readers than a misclassified man or woman.

The inquiry into the "hermaphrodite's" reproductive potential was bound up with concerns about the body politic's health, especially in the French context.[11] Fear of population shrinkage was triggered by repeated wars in the early modern period, monarchical instability, the untimely death of male kings, and the inability of the French monarchy to produce male heirs, which continued well into the eighteenth century, not least because seven years elapsed before Louis XVI and Marie-Antoinette produced offspring (McClive 17–18). While the British did not have the same fears as the French regarding the health of their rulers, they were likewise intent on not only maintaining but also expanding their population in the context of their mercantile and imperial endeavors (Cody 19–20).[12] In the Prussian context, a healthy and fecund citizenry provided subjects for the state's military, thereby ensuring its continued strength. Proposals to alter individual bodies are therefore part of the broader context of securing the health and fecundity of the body politic. In fact, oftentimes "hermaphrodites" were discovered when their marriage remained childless, as was the case with Grandjean. Accused by a former lover of being a "hermaphrodite," Grandjean's wife "reflected on the sterility of their union … and her conscience was alarmed" ["fit des réflexions sur la stérilité de son union … sa conscience fut alarmée"] (Vermeil 7). As a male, Grandjean had been unable to sire children. After surgical intervention to transform him into a woman, Champeaux argued, Grandjean could possibly reproduce. He observes the necessary anatomy for "facilitating the passage of children" ["faciliter le passage des enfants"] (49) and claims that Grandjean's unusual genitalia would not provide an obstacle: "The excessive elongation of the clitoris cannot prevent her from getting married to a man and from having children with him: suppose that it constituted an obstacle, it could easily be amputated, which we have asserted could be achieved without any danger" ["ce prolongement excessif [of the clitoris] ne peut l'empêcher de se marier avec un homme et d'en avoir des enfants: supposé même qu'il format quelque obstacle, il seroit bientôt levé par l'amputation, que nous avons dit pouvoir se faire sans aucun danger"] (54). Champeaux positions the surgeon as the agent who could write a heterosexual ending to the "hermaphrodite's" story. A direct line can be traced from the graphic textual descriptions in the eighteenth century to violent medical interventions that would become the standard of care for individuals with genitals that were considered nonstandard in the second half of the twenty-first century.

Preformationists and Epigenesists

Eighteenth-century physicians' case histories on "hermaphrodites" were embedded in larger debates about reproduction that posed questions about the role of men and women in generating a healthy citizenry. Scientists studying reproduction in the seventeenth and the eighteenth centuries can be divided into two main groups, preformationists and epigenesists. Preformationists believed that a miniature human (homunculus) existed as a preformed entity either in the female egg (ovists) or in male sperm (spermists). By contrast, epigenesists believed that the fetus arose from a process during which two substances merged. Both sides faced considerable difficulties in proving their theory. Epigenesists were at pains to explain the mechanism that led to the creation of a new human being. Preformationists struggled with the explanation of how God could allow either the waste of sperm cells (and the loss of millions of homunculi) or, as Clara Pinto-Correia puts it with respect to the ovists, "the disturbing fact that God had chosen to put His most perfect creation inside the body of a lesser being" (273). The fact that, in the eighteenth century, preformationism was the more dominant theory might appear as a contradiction in an age that purported to illuminate all realms of knowledge with empirical science. However, for many Enlightenment thinkers—including epigenesists—the concept of a rational universe ordered by God was not necessarily seen as a contradiction.

The move away from divine intervention in the natural world was gradual and contested and can be seen in the debates surrounding the terminological shift from "generation" to "reproduction."[13] The word generation implied divine intervention; by contrast, the term reproduction had a more mechanistic connotation. It was first used to describe the reproduction of severed limbs in jellyfish and other invertebrates. Then, the eighteenth-century French natural philosopher Georges-Louis Leclerc Buffon used it to designate human reproduction. From there, it gradually entered scientific discourse, not without opposition from those who wanted to continue emphasizing God's ordering hand. The term reproduction "functioned as a catalyst that could explain structural interrelationships, dynamic change, and natural, rather than religious, causes for life" (Cody 21). The inquiry into these causes aligned with the empirical drive to identify the reasons that led to the birth of individuals with variable sex characteristics. From Antiquity to early modern times, various causes had been proposed for the existence of "hermaphroditic" bodies, ranging from the mother's imagination at the time of conception to God's punishment for moral transgressions.[14] Physicians studying "hermaphrodites" in the eighteenth century strove to move away from these explanatory models.

In their quest to understand "hermaphrodites," medical men focused their examinations on living individuals. Some of them, however, also resorted to dissections, not of dead individuals but of deceased fetuses. Toward the end of his study on Drouart, Ferrein presents the results of such an inquiry:

> I have observed that all female embryos have a penis attached to the pubic bone during the first months of pregnancy; it protrudes and nearly appears like that of male embryos. Those that see them and who are not informed about anatomy customarily believe that they are male; I have seen this happen more than once. Everybody remembers having heard about three- to four-month-old aborted fetuses who, it is said, are nearly all male and rarely female … they indeed appear as such, at first glance.
>
> [J'ai observé que dans les premiers mois de la grossesse tous les embrions femelles ont une verge attachée aux os pubis, saillante & figurée à peu près comme celle des mâles, en sorte que ceux qui les voient sans être au fait de l'Anatomie, ont coutume de les prendre pour tels; c'est ce que j'ai vu arriver plus d'une fois. Chacun peut se rappeler que s'il a entendu parler d'avortons de trois à quatre mois, ces sont presque toujours, dit-on des males, & et rarement des femelles … ils paroissent tels, en effet, au premier coup d'oeil] (339)

Ferrein argues that, at a certain developmental stage, each fetus appears as male because of the presence of a penis-like structure. He claims that "nobody, at least not that I know, has observed what I am reporting" ["personne, au moins que je sache, n'ait observé tout ce que je rapporte"] (339). Two decades earlier, in 1741, however, across the channel, James Parsons had made a similar observation: "All female Foetus's, during the greatest Part of the Time of Gestation, have the Clitoris as large in Proportion to their Sizes, and sometimes larger, than the Angolan Woman before-mentioned" (147). Ferrein and Parsons both hypothesized that this genital structure would eventually lose its ambiguity as the surrounding parts grow and that the fetus would be revealed as female. Both scientists use this observation to argue that there is no such thing as an adult "hermaphrodite," only wrongly categorized women, either in utero or after birth.

By exploring embryonic development, Ferrein and Parsons align themselves with epigenesist rather than preformationist theories. They observe a peculiarity in female embryonic development, described as a penis-like organ by Ferrein and an enlarged clitoris by Parsons. During pregnancy, between week seven and week twelve, the fetus's genitals develop. In week nine, the penis emerges; in weeks eleven and twelve the ovaries develop. The penis and the clitoris remain the same length until week fourteen. In the eighteenth century, these embryonic processes were not yet fully understood. Ferrein and Parsons comment on the stage when penis and clitoris are hard to differentiate. Their observation provides one of the pieces of the complex puzzle of embryonic development that scientists, such as the prominent epigenesist Caspar Friedrich Wolff, began to assemble during the eighteenth century. In 1759, Wolff discovered the ducts from which emerge the external male genitals, which would later be called Wolffian or mesonephric ducts. After nine weeks, the Wolffian ducts gradually regress in the female fetus.[15] Wolff's research in this area opposed him to Haller, one of the most powerful medical men in the eighteenth century and a preformationist.[16] While controversial at their time of publication, Wolff's findings contributed to the gradual replacement of preformation with epigenesis.[17] The idea that embryos developed in stages had significant consequences for understanding sex development. If a female fetus was dissected at a relatively early stage of gestation, it was possible that remnants of the Wolffian ducts were still present, making the fetus appear "hermaphroditic." Parsons and Ferrein might be describing such a fetus in 1740, before Wolff's discovery, and in 1767, a decade later, respectively. Their hypothesizing shows that epigenetic ideas regarding fetal development and sexual differentiation were percolating throughout the century.[18]

Physicians who attempted to frame their explanation of living "hermaphrodites" with an investigation of epigenetic processes in embryos, however, generated more questions than answers. Burghart explicitly thematizes the limits of scientific research, thereby questioning the Enlightenment's focus on empiricism: "How hermaphrodites come into being? … I have to confess in advance that I do not know. Do not be surprised to hear this from an imperial natural scientist. This strikes a blow to the imagined omniscience of scholars … In the end I had more questions than I was given answers and finally, after I had read everything, I knew nothing" ["Woher die Zwitter entstünden? … Denn ich will Ihnen ganz aufrichtig zum voraus bekennen, daß ich es nicht weiß. Nehmen Sie ja keine erstaunende Mine an, solch ein Wort von mir, einem Kaiserli. Naturforscher, zu hören, welches der eingebildeten All- oder doch Viel-Wisserei der Herren Gelehrten, einen so gewaltigen Stoß giebet … Allemal blieb mir noch mehr übrig zu fragen, als man mir beantworten konte, und endlich, nachdem ich alles gelesen hatte, wuste ich so viel als nichts"] (23).

While Burghart seems to accept epistemological uncertainty, other scientists ventured further, literally and figuratively, by turning their attention toward various types of cultural "others" in their construction of the "hermaphrodite." Parsons's case history on the Angolan "hermaphrodite" is the most famous of these investigations. It juxtaposes a dissected fetus with an individual from a remote locale. Through this comparison, Parsons strives to distance himself from cultural locales beyond the European realm in view of enforcing normative behavior at home. As Chapter 4 will show, however, because of the intersectional nature of identities, the distinctions between Europeans and non-Europeans, on the one hand, and men and women, on the other, were muddled as scientists embarked on their imperial scientific journeys. Their reports of these investigations were, in turn, shaped by the narrative conventions of entertainment science with which they positioned themselves in the medical and in the literary marketplace.

Notes

1 On the conception of menstruation in humoral medicine, also see Dean-Jones.

2 In French, the possessive pronoun takes the grammatical gender of the noun it modifies. "Vagin" is masculine in French; therefore, the French pronoun is masculine. As a result, this sentence obscures Hoin's conclusion that Drouart is female.

3 On this point, especially the differences between Galenic/Hippocratic and Aristotelian thinking, also see De Renzi, Hacke, and MacLean.

4 See Matthew Cobb on these seventeenth-century discoveries.

5 The complex relationship between blood and milk in humoral thinking is discussed in Orland. Also see De Renzi for an overview of the differences between Galenic and Aristotelian thinking regarding menstrual blood. While, for Galen, "menstrual blood provided the fetus with nourishment" (De Renzi 209), for Aristotle "conception occurred as a result of the male seed acting upon menstrual blood in the womb" (207). Also see Paster for a broader overview of the body as a humoral entity.

6 Michael Stolberg argues that the plethora model "made periodical bleeding in men as plausible and acceptable as a 'normal' event" ("Menstruation" 96).

7 In "Menstruating Men," Gianna Pomata contends that, at a time when the male body was generally seen as the gold standard, the female body became the standard of comparison when it came to periodical bleeding.

8 A discussion of bloodletting practices in the early modern period can be found in Keller.

9 On the scientific link between menstruation and ovulation, see McClive.

10 Theresa Braunschneider and Valerie Traub discuss the importance ascribed to the clitoris in reproduction during the sixteenth and seventeenth centuries. The focus on the clitoris was a result of the publication of anatomical handbooks, which became possible after the end of the medieval period that was dominated by scholastic writings. The clitoris was considered capable of erection and ejaculation, in analogy to the penis. Female pleasure therefore was seen as central to the reproductive process in the early modern period.

11 See Blum and Tuttle on the connection between the body and the body politic with respect to reproduction.

12 On eighteenth-century concerns about insufficient population growth, also see Schiebinger, *Plants and Empire* 234–5.

13 On this topic, see Stephanson and Wagner, *The Secrets of Generation.*

14 In her *Gender, Pregnancy, and Power in Eighteenth-Century Literature*, Jenifer Buckley discusses eighteenth-century thinking regarding the role of the maternal imagination in the process of generation.

15 It is now known that this regression is the result of a complex process that involves sex chromosomes, protein, hormones, and the activation of a gene network (Wizemann and Pardue).

16 Haller had actually started out as an epigenesist, yet he espoused preformationism sometime between 1740 and 1755. Preformationism allowed him to posit an ordering master in the form of God. On this point see Pinto-Correia and Shirley Roe. For a discussion of the tension between empiricism and the persisting desire for transcendental meaning in the eighteenth century, see Poovey.

17 Questioning an influential man such as Haller made it difficult for Wolff to find work in the close-knit European medical community. After working as a surgeon in the Prussian army, he gave private lectures to paying students before moving to a permanent position in Saint Petersburg (Aulie 124–44).

18 Only in 1830 would the paramesonephric system—which develops into the fallopian tubes, uterus, and the upper part of the vagina—be discovered and described by Johannes Peter Müller.

4

Terra Incognita/Parts Unknown

The German scientist Gottfried Heinrich Burghart seemed to accept the fact that he had more questions than answers after having read the published material on the topic of "hermaphroditism." In his *Gründliche Nachricht an seinen Freund **** (1763), he even appeared to relish the epistemological aporia that, at its core, questioned the Enlightenment project to understand and classify every aspect of the natural world. It was the inability to find conclusive answers that kept the issue of "hermaphroditism" alive and thereby allowed physicians to benefit financially and professionally. Typically without any other means of subsistence, individuals who were labeled "hermaphrodites" eked out a living by roaming the European medical landscape, appealing not only to an academic audience but also to a rapidly growing reading public interested in popularizing accounts of scientific, including medical, topics. Medical men assumed that additional and more detailed examinations of individual "hermaphrodites" would provide more conclusive answers. In their quest for more information, they turned to exotic locales that figured prominently in the eighteenth-century imagination. Remote territories that European nations were in the process of exploring and exploiting economically played a central role in the way sex and gender were imagined during this time period.

While Michel Foucault's work has been crucial for understanding eighteenth-century sexuality in general and "hermaphroditism" in particular, it largely neglects the impact of European imperialism and colonialism on these particular issues. Responding to Foucault's work, Ann Laura Stoler argues that "Europe's eighteenth-century discourses on sexuality can—indeed must—be traced along a more *circuitous imperial* route" (7; emphasis in original). This imperial route is explored neither in Foucault's four-volume *History of Sexuality*, nor in his other writings on sexuality such as *Les anormaux*, which explicitly discuss "hermaphrodites." Stoler is not the only one to note the lack of scholarship exploring the intersection of Enlightenment thought with (post) colonialism. In their introduction to the *Social Text* issue on the biopolitics of plasticity, Kyla Schuller and Jules Gill-Peterson underscore the fact that Foucault's concept of biopolitical racism largely ignores the transatlantic slave trade and colonialism. In addition, Daniel Carey and Lynn Festa remark that "none of the major studies—Cassirer, Gay, Foucault, Horkheimer and Adorno—explicitly analyses the colonial projects of the eighteenth century, while recent accounts of Counter-Enlightenment … barely glance at the postcolonial critique of Enlightenment" (17–18). As a result, there has not been a long-standing and robust dialogue between eighteenth-century studies and analyses of European colonial projects. Therefore, approaches to texts from this time period often miss the multiple intersections between European colonialism and other realities, such as class and gender, that shaped collective and individual identities.

Analyzing the circuitous imperial paths that connect gender and sexuality in the emerging global world is, however, crucial in order to uncover those ambiguities that are not explored in Thomas Laqueur's posited shift from the one- to the two-sex model in the eighteenth century. Laqueur, who largely adopts a Foucauldian line of argumentation, highlights the sixteenth and seventeenth centuries' struggle with the meaning of the discovery of foreign territories for the conceptualization of sex and gender. In his discussion of the eighteenth century, however, the analysis of the imperial context is notably absent. In this respect, Laqueur's approach is symptomatic for academic discussions of the eighteenth century. Wedged in-between the early explorations of the sixteenth and seventeenth centuries and full-fledged colonialism in the nineteenth century, the eighteenth century often figures as an afterthought in scholarship. As Dorinda Outram has argued poignantly, eighteenth-century scholars "have yet to come to grips with the relation between the Enlightenment and the creation of a global world" (3). Exploring the intertwinement of sexuality with imperialism during this time period is crucial because of the "historically unprecedented establishment of exploitative power relations with non-European people on a global scale" (Wheeler 11). These power relations profoundly affected every aspect of Europeans' life, not only abroad but also at home.[1]

Imperial Commodification

With the establishment of teaching hospitals and the commodification of medical knowledge, scientists had increased access to bodies that did not fit existing norms on the European continent. When their examinations of domestic "hermaphrodites" did not yield definitive results, they turned their attention to faraway places, duplicating the exploitative power relations that rendered possible medical inquiries at home. Imperial subjects became overdetermined signifiers in discussions about sex and gender. They were commodified in a trade network that extended from the medical realm to the popular book market. "Hermaphrodites" thereby embodied the three interconnected themes of emerging Western imperialism in the eighteenth century: "The transmission of white, male power through control of colonized women; the emergence of a new global order of cultural knowledge; and the imperial command of commodity capital" (McClintock 2–3).

James Parsons's *A Mechanical and Critical Enquiry into the Nature of Hermaphrodites* (1741) is the most famous text illustrating the three elements of this male, imperial, and commercialized epistemology. In scholarship, Parsons's *Enquiry* typically figures as the text that, in the first part of the eighteenth century, moved individuals with variable sex characteristics from the mythological to the scientific realm by conclusively arguing that there are no human "hermaphrodites" but only mis-categorized men or women. The *Enquiry*'s stated goal is the description of a dissected fetus with ambiguous genitals, about whom Parsons does not provide any additional information. As discussed extensively in Chapter 1, this description, however, is only presented in the conclusion of Parsons's treatise and is preceded by a historical survey of previous literature on "hermaphroditism" that ranges from Greek and Roman thinkers such as Empedocles, Parmenides, and Augustine to the seventeenth-century scientists Ambroise Paré, Regnier de Graaf, and Isbrand van Diemerbroeck. While Parsons's reference points are European scholars and a presumably European fetus, the impetus for writing the *Enquiry* is the result of the imperial context, as he points out in the preface: "The Arrival of the *Angolan Woman* in Town encouraged this undertaking … which rendered it not an unseasonable Time to make a further Progress in this Essay" (liv; emphasis in original). The presence of the Angolan in the center of London signals British imperial power and explores the profitable marketplace for exotic curiosities. For the price of nearly three shillings, the curious could view this imperial subject and, for approximately the same amount, they could purchase Parsons's treatise (Fontes da Costa 132–3). The Enlightenment project of classifying the natural world coincided with imperialism and was dependent on it, making the year 1741 "not an unseasonable time" for Parsons to publish a treatise on "hermaphroditism."

Parsons mentions the "Arrival of the *Angolan Woman* in Town" to explain the genesis of his *Enquiry*. In the main body of the treatise, Parsons provides more information about the provenance of his object of study: "This woman was carried from Angola in Africa, amongst other Slaves, to America, from whence she was brought to Bristol" (134). From there, the Angolan was transported to London and put on display. In one sentence, Parsons condenses the realities of the slave trade triangle that connected the African continent, England, and Caribbean and North American plantations, hiding the responsibility of the colonizer by using the passive voice ("was carried"). Rather than remaining on an American plantation, however, the Angolan enters the British homeland through the same port city—Bristol—from which many British ships departed on their triangular journey. The Angolan's journey from Africa to America and then to Europe via Bristol encapsulates the realities of the mid-eighteenth-century slave trade. The Angolan's journey began as a field or domestic laborer but concluded as a commodity in the marketplace for entertainment science. These different types of marketplaces were connected in a network that was based on the exchange of human bodies and goods across vast geographical and cultural divides.

Bristol had been a key location for British imperial expansion. Situated on the rivers Avon and Frome, it became the leading British port over the course of the first decades of the eighteenth century. As a result, Bristol changed from a medieval town to a bustling imperial marketplace. From Bristol, British manufactured goods (and those imported from East India) were shipped to West Africa. From West Africa, mainly Angola, slaves were transported to Caribbean and North American territories. Vessels then carried raw materials, predominately coffee, sugar and tobacco, back to Bristol, from where they entered the European marketplace and went into distribution for processing into luxury consumer goods. During the 1730s and 1740s, it became more perilous for Bristol ships to reach the African coast because of the Wars of Austrian Succession and resulting privateering ventures of other European imperial powers.[2] This, in turn, made it financially riskier for Bristol merchants to embark on the long journey, which could take an entire year to complete. Bristol's importance as a port city began to decline in the mid-eighteenth century and it was soon overtaken by Liverpool.[3] As a result, Bristol merchants' profits began to shrink, leading to severe credit problems due to non-collected remittances. In the context of these developments, the 1741 import of the Angolan slave into the British homeland via Bristol carries particular significance.

Spectacular Suffering

At a time when Bristol merchants experienced financial losses on investments in their traditional realm of business, exhibiting a slave as a "hermaphrodite" positioned their commercial ventures in the marketplace for both exotic and anatomical curiosities. The revenue from exhibiting the Angolan might have been used to appease impatient and dissatisfied investors. Palmira Fontes da Costa summarizes the intense marketing of the exhibit of the Angolan slave after being transported to the center of the British empire, London:

> Advertisements of an African hermaphrodite appeared regularly in London newspapers throughout 1741. For the price of two shillings and sixpence the "Famous African" was to be seen at the Golden Cross, near Charring Cross, from nine in the morning until three in the afternoon, and from four in the afternoon until ten at night up some stairs in the corner of the Little Piazza, Covent Garden. (129)

The locations of this exhibit are significant in several respects. A square in London created by the intersection of several streets, Charing Cross was a transportation hub which connected the capital to numerous British cities such as Bristol, but also Brighton, Bath, Cambridge, Dover, and York. In addition, Charing Cross was the place where executions were carried out and criminals were flogged. Numerous taverns bordered the square and made it a prime location for popular entertainment venues.[4] A hub for commerce and entertainment during the day, Charing Cross was a strategic choice for the exhibit of the Angolan from the morning to the early afternoon. One advertisement explicitly states the exhibit's easy accessibility by mentioning that "Here is a Coach-Way from St. Martin's-Lane to the Stairs-Foot" (*London Daily*, January 15, 1741). From the late afternoon to the late evening, the Angolan was moved to an area in Covent Garden. Covent Garden was the site not only of the renowned opera, built in 1732 and mainly used for Handel's performances, but also of the red-light district that housed some of the most (in)famous eighteenth-century prostitutes.

Both London sites—Charing Cross and Covent Garden—demonstrate the intertwinement of business, culture, and (sexual) entertainment. The connections between these three realms create what Ramesh Mallipeddi has called "spectacular suffering," which establishes "the problem of slavery as a problem of embodiment" (3). In the advertisements, the Angolan is never described as a slave but is strategically called the "Famous African" or "Native Angolan" in a way that generated interest without openly alienating those critical of slavery, the numbers of which were growing during this time period. At the same that the Angolan's body is at the center of these exhibits, their individuality is erased due to the absence of a name, projecting them into the realm of total alterity and, to borrow a term from postcolonial criticism, subalternity. The public exhibit ran for ten consecutive months. In addition, displays occurred at private residences, which underlines the popularity of the exhibit and hints at the considerable revenue that must have been generated by it. The advertisements never mention the recipient of the admission fees, yet it most likely was a slave merchant, potentially from Bristol, who commodified the Angolan not on a North American plantation but in London public spaces and private homes.

Advertisements for the exhibit of the Angolan appeared in such publications as *The London Daily Post and General Advertiser*. The advertisements are located among classifieds and news that themselves repeatedly reference the era's colonial context. In addition to real estate notices, advertisements for chimney vents, and declarations of bankruptcies, the *London Daily* reports on the value of South Sea bonds, Jamaican rum, and ships departing for places in Britain's growing empire. Interspersed amid news of Britain's commercial ventures are reports for medical cures for diseases such as scurvy that were the direct result of the imperial context or for sexually transmitted diseases like syphilis that spread and mutated as Europeans traveled to regions far away from home.[5] Cures for cancer also figure prominently among these classifieds, often triggered by the hope of discovering new remedies in faraway lands. Londa Schiebinger posits this "bioprospecting" as a central component of the "Atlantic World Medical Complex" (*Secret Cures* 3), which she describes as "three major nexuses across which people and their knowledges moved: the colonial nexus linking Europe and the Americas, the slave trade nexus joining Africa and the Americas, and the conquest nexus that brought Amerindian practices into the plantation complex" (13). The intersection of these three elements with developments in the medical sphere and the publishing realm commodified the Angolan as a good to be marketed and consumed in the eighteenth-century marketplace for science-as-entertainment.

Consumer Goods

In March 1741, after ten consecutive months of intense interest, the marketing strategy changed, presumably because of declining interest and, consequently, revenue. First, viewing hours were shortened to 3 p.m. In May 1741, the hours were extended again, until 10 p.m.; this time, however, the Angolan was displayed in only one location, Charing Cross, and the price was reduced to "no more than 1 s. each" (*London Daily*, May 2). In addition to the price reduction, the advertisements create a sense of urgency—"our Stay here being but short" (*London Daily*, March 24) and "For the small Time we stay here" (*London Daily*, May 2)—with the goal of attracting paying customers. Viewers were also lured to the exhibit with the promise of printed material that could be taken home. The March advertisement mentions that a "particular Description of the Parts which distinguish the Sexes, is in the Hand Bills, and likewise it will be given at the Place" (*London Daily*, March 24), presumably without any additional charge. Similarly, the May advertisement states that "at this Place only may be had a curious engraved Figure taken from, and as big as the Life, done by the ingenious Mr. Vandergucht, at 1 s. each, to be Sold to none but those who have seen or come to view the Original" (*London Daily*, May 2). The printed material was no longer available for free but could be purchased; moreover, the purchase was limited to those also paying for the exhibit. The illustration, a central piece in many case histories on "hermaphrodites," is presented as a rare commodity and its price is justified by the reference to the artist, Gerard van der Gucht. Gucht was the illustrator of one of the most famous anatomy textbooks of the period, William Cheselden's *Anatomy of the Human Body* (1713), a new edition of which was coincidentally advertised on the same page as the exhibit of the Angolan in the *London Daily's* February 6 issue. The advertised "curious engraved figure" appears to have been the one included in the sixth edition of Cheselden's *Anatomy* (1741) and referenced explicitly in the March 24 advertisement, which also mentions two additional medical authorities, James Douglas, a prominent Scottish surgeon and anatomist, and John Freak, surgeon at St. Bartholomew's hospital in London. Douglas pronounces the Angolan female, Freak considers the Angolan male, and Cheselden views the Angolan as a "wonderful Mixture of both Sexes" (*London Daily*, March 24). In addition to imparting a scientific aura to the exhibit, referencing these three medical authorities strategically presented the Angolan as an unsolvable anatomical riddle, thereby keeping the audience's interest alive and their purses open.

The final strategy for broadening the appeal of the exhibit was to target female viewers who, out of concerns regarding its supposed indecency, might have been kept away from Charing Cross. The March 24 and May 2 advertisements state that "Ladies will be attended by a prudent Person of their own Sex." The presence of a female guide was supposed to lessen the potential shock of viewing the "famous African" who, in January, was advertised with the alliterative phrase "Mas, Mulier, Maurus; Mundi mirabile Monstrum! ["Manly woman, Moor; the world's marvelous wonder"].[6] The use of Latin both sensationalized the exhibit and strove to give it an academic appearance through the de facto exclusion of those unversed in the language of science, such as women and people from socially and economically disadvantaged strata of society. The reduced price of admission at Charing Cross and the advertised moral guidance, however, made the Angolan accessible to both groups. Never having been given a name that recognized their humanity, the Angolan was further objectified when they were eventually moved from London to York for display during the town's horse races as a result of the capitalist logic of the eighteenth-century entertainment marketplace.[7]

Female Consumption

Exhibitors' targeting of female viewers in their advertisements highlights the ambivalent position of women in eighteenth-century consumer culture. Typically excluded from any type of business ventures in the imperial context, upper-class women were the prime consumers of exotic imports such as tea, coffee, and chocolate. Elizabeth Kowaleski-Wallace has detailed the complex ways in which the tea table functioned in the eighteenth century, with respect to both gender and class. Consumption of those imports signified social standing, enabling the aristocracy to cement their social relevance and making it possible for merchants, who were accumulating significant wealth during this time, to climb the social ladder and set themselves apart from the lower classes.

The female body became an ambivalent signifier in these shifting networks where the meaning of "consumption" encompassed both the mercantile and the medical realm.[8] On the one hand, consumption of luxury goods signified wealth and refinement, as represented in the pale and fainting bodies of many eighteenth-century protagonists. On the other, however, these consumptive episodes also signified a dangerous weakening of life forces in women and therefore crystallized the fears of the particular social stratum to which they belonged. The female body, responsive to external stimuli, was seen as fluid and therefore uncontrollable and ultimately threatening: "Fluidity, we might say, has come to be associated with the threat of woman as other—the danger of a potentially controlled dispersion that cannot be fixed in place, that seeps through 'the cracks in the overall system'" (Salvaggio 26).[9] Woman's supposed fluidity was further increased by her consumption of those fluids symptomatic of imperial success, such as coffee, tea, and hot chocolate, whose properties contemporaries were still in the process of exploring.

The fear of the female body was displaced onto the figure of the "hermaphrodite." In turn, investigations of "hermaphroditic" bodies led, not surprisingly, to subjects outside the domestic context: "Rapidly expanding consumer practices in the West occurred against the backdrop of colonial expansion, bringing the British consumer into contact with her dark sister, the underimagined female Caribbean slave, whose labors would help fuel the British economy" (Kowaleski-Wallace 147). The Angolan "hermaphrodite" functions like the Caribbean female slave by contributing to the British marketplace for medical knowledge and salacious entertainment. The fact that the Angolan, rather than staying on a North American plantation, had to labor in the British homeland, literalizes the interpenetration of the domestic and the foreign. Exploring the imperial route is therefore crucial for understanding eighteenth-century discourses on sexuality and their intertwinement with emerging and consolidating concepts of race.

Women as "Hermaphrodites?"

The Angolan embodies the "cross-hatched representations of race, gender, and anomaly" (*The Limits of the Human* 1) discussed by Felicity Nussbaum. The Angolan's "defective and racialized femininity … paradoxically energizes an imperial England as it struggles to demarcate the limits of the human through women" (2). The Angolan's ultimate display at the horse races in York is significant in this context as it juxtaposes them with nonhuman, animal life forms. The alignment of "hermaphroditism" with an aberrant humanity and racialized femininity is emphasized in the advertisements of the Angolan exhibit: "Mas, Mulier, Maurus; Mundi mirabile Monstrum!" The Angolan is described as a "manly woman," a "moor," and a "monster." The use of Latin purports to hide the salacious content at the same time that it sensationalizes it. In addition, employing Latin echoes eighteenth-century classification systems, most famously represented by Carl Linnaeus's *Systema Naturae* (1735). The subtitle of the *Systema* summarizes Linnaeus's taxonomic project as a "system of nature through the three kingdoms of nature, according to classes, orders, genera and species, with characters, differences, synonyms, places."[10] Linnaeus set out to categorize the entirety of the natural world in a system of Latin binomial taxonomy, in which the first part designates the genus and the second the species.

In the five-page-long captions that accompany the *Enquiry*'s illustrations, Parsons uses Latin to present the Angolan as a woman, albeit one with uncommon genitals. In his search for the most appropriate terminology to describe the external genitals, Parsons, like Linnaeus, uses binomial terms and vacillates between "*Nympha Luxurians*" and "*Clytoris, magnitudine aucta*" before settling on "the true *Nympha Muliebris*" (136). While the first two terms emphasize the clitoris's and labia's supposedly unusual size—"luxurians" and "magnitudine aucta"—and thereby open room for a discussion of its bearer's sex, the third term positions the Angolan unequivocally as a woman; as "muliebris." Even though Parsons acknowledges the *Nymphae Mulibieris*' "uncommon Length and Bigness" (136), he immediately negates the possibility that the labia—by which he seemingly means the clitoris—could be a penis by claiming that it had "not the smallest Perforation or Opening" (136). The binomial structure "Nymphae mulibieris" mimics Linnean terminology, aligning the clitoris with exotic flowers imported to Europe for study by famous botanists. Londa Schiebinger argues that "Botanical Latin" (*Plants and Empire* 20) was intimately tied to the construction of the scientist's "heroic masculinity" (65). Parsons presents himself as the one who, with the tools and the language of empirical science, can solve the mystery of nonbinary sex and ultimately classify it away. Like Linnaeus, Parsons never crossed the Atlantic; the interconnected networks of imperial commerce and science ensured that the most memorable specimens landed on the European scientist's desk without him ever having to leave home. Empiricism and imperialism were mutually constitutive in the eighteenth century's epistemological networks.

Climate

Exotic goods, botanical specimens, and humans entered European homes and research spaces in various forms. The *Enquiry*'s intent was to prove that all supposed "hermaphrodites" were merely women with an overdeveloped clitoris and that those women occur with greater frequency in equatorial territories:

> We have so very few Instances among the European Nations of those so reputed; though, as is before observed, they are common enough in Africa and Asia, in all those Places especially that are nearest the Equinoctial Line; where the Nonnaturals themselves conduce much to the general

> Relaxation of the Solids, and consequently, this unseemly Accretion of that Part. (Parsons 147)

Parsons opposes European bodies to those in a warmer climate, which was thought to cause a "general relaxation of the solids" that could lead to an overdeveloped clitoris. By contrasting the Angolan with domestic subjects, Parsons engages emerging climate theories that were gradually replacing humoral notions of the body. Climate was seen to affect the individual's body and was used to hierarchize different populations:

> In the eighteenth century, proximity to Europe and to temperate climates generated a theoretical hierarchy … that placed Europeans, and a few groups from the Middle East and North Africa, at the top and Africans and Laplanders at the bottom. Because of the excessive heat that was believed to enervate the body, mind and morals, commonplaces about the torrid zone being the home of dark-skinned people who were indolent, lascivious, and subject to tyranny often seemed confirmed when Englishmen confronted social and political life as well as labor arrangements that were alien to them. (Wheeler 24)

Moderate climate was interpreted in a favorable light, whereas heat was thought to affect the body and the mind in a negative way.[11] With this interpretation, Europeans sought to make sense of the realities they encountered in the territories they were exploring. The result was what Mark Harrison calls a "medico-climactic discourse … [that] was commonly invoked in order to account for the dynamism of European culture and the increasing dominance of European over Asian states" (59) and, one might add, the African continent.

At the same time that climate theory established an opposition between Europe and Africa/Asia, it also contained the seeds for questioning this same binary. Climate theory meant that humans were shaped by the environment and, by extension, could adapt to it. This adaptability was important in the context of Europeans' forays into "the torrid zone," a term used since Aristotle to refer to the equatorial regions.[12] The less attached thinkers were to the idea of biological immutability, the more optimistic they were about the feasibility of the colonial project. Because people could adapt to different climates, Europeans and Africans were not viewed as diametrically opposite—as they were in the biologically essentialist racial thinking of the nineteenth century—but were thought to possess commonalities. In this view of, what Ivan Hannaford has described as a pre-idea of race, the human body was a malleable entity with porous borders. At the same time that climate theory made it possible to imagine successful colonization of tropical regions, it also posed the question of what this adaptability meant for the European body. In the context of the British colonization of India, Mark Harrison observes that "many Europeans continued to believe that human character (and even physical appearance) could be shaped by the environment, so that Europeans might eventually become 'Indianized' by long residence on the subcontinent" (60). At the same time that this thinking allowed Europeans to be optimistic about their potential for success in the imperial context, it also caused anxiety, especially with respect to European women, whose bodies were seen as particularly fluid and who could evade the control of their fathers, husbands, and brothers. The cult of domesticity, propagated in fiction and conduct manuals, was a direct result of the fear of losing control of the domestic woman in an imperial context.[13] Felicity Nussbaum explores how the "invention of the 'other' woman of empire enabled the consolidation of the cult of domesticity in England and, at the same time, the association of the sexualized woman at home with the exotic, or 'savage,' non-European woman" (*Torrid Zones* 1). The foreign woman was both different and the same as the domestic one.

The notion that inhabitants of the torrid zone were lascivious permeated eighteenth-century discussions of African women. The prominent French naturalist George-Louis Leclerc Buffon "was clearly fascinated by portraits of beautiful hypersexual African women … On the one hand, Buffon suggested that the African woman's body was closer than the European woman's body to its primal function. … On the other hand, Buffon believed that the excessive debauchery that supposedly defined an African woman's life left an indelible mark on her body" (Andrew Curran 112), such as an elongated clitoris. The African woman was simultaneously more and less of a woman because her body was visibly marked by her supposed exuberant sexuality. The framing of African femininity as fertile yet monstrous occurred in the context of a change in thinking about explored territories. This change is reflected in the shift in terminology from the "torrid zone," which had been used since classical antiquity to refer to the hot regions of the earth, to the "tropics," which invoked both fecundity and decay (Harrison 59). In the context of climate theory, the African woman's supposed hypersexuality was a result of her habitat; European women were therefore not immune to becoming like their African or Indian sisters, especially not if they moved to the same geographical area. Parsons invokes the Angolan to establish a clear demarcation between foreign and domestic, yet the binary that he so carefully seeks to establish has cracks. Those cracks appear when he observes that "we have so very few Instances among the European Nations of those so reputed; though, as is before observed, they are common enough in Africa and Asia" (147). Rather than claiming that there are no women with supposedly overdeveloped genitals in Europe, Parsons states that there are "very few," unable to exclude their existence in the domestic realm. Ultimately, *all* female sexuality is potentially aberrant and threatening.

Because race was a fluid concept in the eighteenth century, Parsons's attempt to use it to consolidate sexual difference posed questions instead of foreclosing them. The pre-idea of race resembled the one-sex model, which had not yet been completely supplanted by the two-sex model. Both interpretive frameworks positioned humans on a continuum rather than in a binary structure, allowing for gradual transitions and intersections in identity with respect to sex and race. The fact that Parsons describes the mass in the Angolan's hernia as either an "ovarium or testicle" (137) points at his own indecision and aligns him with the one-sex model, which described these anatomical structures as "stones," preceded by the qualifier "male" or "female." Even though Parsons strives to establish the Angolan as a woman and to uphold the binary, the Angolan functions as a "hermaphrodite" in his text. In fact, the framing of the Angolan with an "enquiry into the nature of hermaphrodites" and the dissemination of the text in the marketplace for entertainment science reifies the medical category of "hermaphroditism" at the same time that Parsons seeks to dismantle it. Despite all statements to the contrary, Parsons's description of the racial other's physique did not provide the expected clarity on sexual difference. Conversely, sexuality operated as an ambivalent signifier in the attempt to understand the differences in people from different geographical regions.

Buffon's comment about African women's hypersexuality was part of a broader inquiry into the varieties of people in the eighteenth century. Two main theories competed for prominence; both of those sought to replace biblical with scientific explanations: monogenesis and polygenesis. Buffon was the most prominent representative of monogenesis. Monogenesis posited a common origin for all humans and was, in a sense, aligned with the biblical story of Adam (Aderibigbe 26).[14] Polygenesis, whose most famous proponent was Voltaire, established the most radical break with the scriptures as it postulated different ancestors for people from different geographical areas: "At the heart of the polygenetic position was a refusal to believe that other people who appeared in every way 'savage' and physically different could be from the same ancestors. This was particularly the case if Europeans compared themselves to Africans" (Horsman 48). Monogenesis' conclusions could have been more egalitarian than those of polygenesis; its implications, however, overlapped with those of polygenetic thinkers because monogenesis considered the different races to be the result of a gradual process of degeneration from a common white ancestor (Andrew Curran 118). Monogenesists used the example of the Black albino as proof for their theory. The monogenesist Pierre Louis Maupertius argued that, since "there were only *nègres blancs* and no *blancs nègres* … the white variety was clearly the forerunner variety from which the black race originated, and to which it sometimes reverted when an albino was born" (Andrew Curran 94). An albino rendered visible the hidden history of white and Black people in the form of a common ancestral origin, which was thought to be white.[15] In scientific discourse, the role played by the African "hermaphrodite" paralleled that of the human albino, especially in debates concerning reproduction. Scientists investigated both as exceptions that could prove the rule in their writing of natural history. The "hermaphrodite" became a privileged signifier in the quest to understand both sexual and racial difference.

The intersectional nature of race and sex came to bear on the hierarchy that established the relative position of different racial and ethnic groups. In this respect, the genitals were not the sole physical markers used to hierarchize groups of individuals, as Londa Schiebinger has shown in her discussion of eighteenth-century anatomical illustrations:

> Anatomists attempted to rank the sexes and races in a single, hierarchical chain of being according to cranium and pelvis size … In respect to skull size, the European male represented the fully developed human type, outranking the African male, the European female, and the African female. In this racial and sexual hierarchy, the European male clearly held the superior position. The relative position of the African male and the European female, however, was not clear-cut. (*The Mind* 211)

Moving from anatomists' discussion of skull circumference to their descriptions of pelvis size, Schiebinger argues that the "inconclusiveness that had plagued the relative position of the African male and European female in relation to cranial capacity was felt here in relation to the position of the African female and European male" (212). When considered together, race and sex produced an ambivalent space on this scale. The figure of the Angolan "hermaphrodite" embodied both types of ambivalence. This ambivalence would gradually disappear in the nineteenth century with the emergence of theories that promoted an essentialist view of race and biology. In the eighteenth century, however, the Angolan "hermaphrodite" still represented the fluid relation between, on the one hand, men and women and, on the other, Africans and Europeans. This instability of racial and sexual categories generated signified anxiety in medical discourse and led to the eventual medicalization of both Black and female bodies.[16]

Surgery and the *Fricatrice*

In contrast to the majority of his seventeenth- and eighteenth-century colleagues, Parsons approvingly describes the reduction or removal of the clitoris practiced be "Asiaticks" and "Africans," more specifically "Egyptians" and "Ethiopians." Rather than characterizing this practice as barbaric, as was customary in the eighteenth-century medical realm, Parsons praises it:

> it is matter of no small surprise, that Authors never were able to take the least hint from the Practice of the People of some of the *Asiatick*, as well as the *African* nations, concerning these large Clitorides … the People knowing that the Length of them produces two Evils, *viz.* the hindering the Coitus, and Women abuse of them with each other, wisely cut or burn them off while Girls are young, and at the same time never entertain the least Notion of the Existence of any other Nature besides the Female in those Subject who are thus depriv'd of that useless Part. (10–11; emphasis in original)

In contrast to many of his contemporaries, Parsons does not present female circumcision of "large Clitorides" as a sign of the cultural other's need for Europe's civilizing intervention. On the contrary, he depicts this practice as a model worth emulating, which is in line with the eighteenth century's devaluing of female sexual pleasure, in the context of reproduction and beyond. Parsons thereby strategically aligns himself with developments in the realm of surgery. Surgeons' firsthand experience and violent manipulation of the human body was increasingly valued in an era focused on empirical knowledge; surgeons were typically consulted to diagnose genitals that were perceived as ambiguous, often in a legal context. Surgery was an assertion of male power, especially in a professional context where male medical practitioners increasingly replaced midwives. While there are very few reports of eighteenth-century surgeons removing or reducing the size of the clitoris, surgical intervention to ensure heterosexual reproduction was not unheard of at this time.[17]

Surgeons functioned as normalizing agents in the service of heterosexual reproductive intercourse; their diagnoses and procedures strove to erase the existence of "confricatrices" (12) or "fricatrices," literally translated as "rubbing women," which were sometimes also called "tribades." Large clitorises were thought to encourage masturbation and same-sex encounters. Eighteenth-century discussions of the "fricatrice" and the "tribade" voiced the fear of self-sufficient female sexuality. Valerie Traub argues that these figures became metonymic of every woman's illicit desire (98). Every woman, independent of her genital anatomy, was potentially a *fricatrice*, undermining her reproductive mission in the enjoyment of her own body or that of other women. Female pleasure became increasingly suspect over the course of the eighteenth century. Whereas it had been considered necessary for reproduction in the sixteenth and seventeenth centuries, it was gradually devalued.[18] Felicity Nussbaum points out that the clitoris "was a particularly vexing body part in the eighteenth century because of its refusal to remain within the feminine domain. It threatened national security and the body politic" (*Torrid Zones* 102). Parsons's suggestion to surgically reduce the size of the clitoris of supposed "hermaphrodites" needs to be read in this context. It had implications for all women because the perception that the clitoris was a potentially "useless part" (Parsons 11) would become more widespread during the eighteenth and especially the nineteenth centuries. Parsons's comment that the Angolan "has often been lain with by Men" (135) points at his work in the service of heteronormative and reproductive sexuality. The passive voice in this sentence thinly veils the violence wielded on the Angolan's body by the realities of slavery, which resulted in the erasure of the Angolan's embodied experience.

Dissecting the Fetus

The intersection of racial and sexual categories in Parsons's description of the Angolan is further complicated by his dissection report on a fetus with ambiguous genitalia, which was the presumable focus of his treatise. While the relation between the fetus and the Angolan "hermaphrodite" appears tangential, their juxtaposition is far from coincidental in an era that valued classification and hierarchization. Only on the last pages of his *Enquiry*, after a lengthy summary of previous writings on "hermaphroditism," does Parsons eventually include the description of the dissected fetus announced in the preface:

> This Subject was an abortive Foetus of about six Months Growth … All female Fœtus's, during the greatest Part of the Time of Gestation, have the Clitoris as large in Proportion to their Sizes, and sometimes larger, than the *Angolan* Woman before-mentioned … Nor is it's [*sic*] Largeness in a Fœtus much to be wondered at, since there are other very similar Cases in the same Body, as the Gland *Thymus* and *Glandulæ Renales* … I opened the above-mentioned Foetus … to manifest the Existence of an Uterus in every Macroclitoridea … it is obvious, what was the Sex of this Subject, without any further Observations on it. (148–54; emphasis in original)

The development of the genitals in the womb was of great scientific interest as it provided clues about epigenetic processes and promised to contribute insights to debates regarding sex and gender. As discussed in Chapter 3, for Parsons, the clitoris functioned as an example of how, during the process of gestation, body parts grow, sometimes disproportionately. He posits that the clitoris is not alone in this respect and cites the renal and thymus glands. Parsons argues that a cursory glance at the outside genitals might indicate either male or ambiguous sex, but that a dissection reveals the presence of a uterus and therefore female sex. He concludes that the excessive development of the clitoris is the result of a particular gestational stage rather than an indicator of the sex at birth.

Parsons's argument about the fetus intersects with his observations about the Angolan "hermaphrodite" in multiple ways. His reference to the exhibited Angolan serves as a strategic springboard for his discussion of the fetus. At the same time, however, his comments on the fetus also serve to elucidate the Angolan's biology. In this context, epigenetic thinking provided a model not only for individual but also for group development and thereby dovetailed with debates about the origins of different racial groups. Parsons implies that, in the same way that a six-month-old fetus is an underdeveloped baby, the Angolan is an underdeveloped adult. In this respect, the oversized clitoris signifies incomplete maturation in a context where different racial and national groups were positioned in relation to one another on a civilizational time line. Whites—Europeans—were placed at the top of this hierarchy, while people of color occupied the bottom. Within each group, there existed an internal order that was determined not only by their skin color but also by their cultural and scientific achievement—hence the inadequateness of the term "race" in the eighteenth century.[19] For some thinkers, like the geographer and diplomat Cornelius de Pauw, "nègres seemed forever stuck in the initial and unfortunate stage of human development; they were ensnared in a 'childhood' or 'original state' that would prevent them from civilizing themselves" (Andrew Curran 127). Parsons's description of the Angolan can be read in this context. While de Pauw's argument relates to African cultural achievements, Parsons discusses the Angolan's anatomy. The adult Angolan's overdeveloped clitoris parallels that of a fetus; the implication of that juxtaposition was that the Angolan had undergone a sort of arrested development and had therefore never reached full maturity. At the same time, however, the enlarged clitoris suggested a degree of hypersexualization that fascinated thinkers like Buffon. This excessive sexuality seemingly contradicted the notion of Africans' perpetual childishness; however, both were closely aligned in discourses on sex and race as they signaled proximity to nature and therefore abundant fertility. The Angolan's body was both dis-abled and extra-abled when it came to their reproductive potential.

Social and Economic Conditions

Parsons's discussion of "hermaphroditism" occurs through the prism of the racial other. In his quest for answers, he juxtaposed sexual and racial alterity with a different kind, in the form of what we nowadays call class, that is a group of people sharing similar social and economic conditions. In his *Enquiry*, Parsons includes an illustration by his mentor, James Douglas, one of the most important eighteenth-century anatomists. In this illustration, race and class intersect because Douglas juxtaposed the Angolan woman's genitals with two illustrations of a "Girl Shewed about Town for an Hermaphrodite" (140).[20] Parsons's large foldout of Douglas's original presents these three genital areas as if they were part of one single body.[21] Only the captions make it clear that these genitals actually belong to two different individuals. The first genital area is that of the Angolan woman and the other two are illustrations of the genitals of the girl shown about town, presumably London. While no further information is given about this individual, they—like most domestic "hermaphrodites"—in all probability were economically disadvantaged and exhibited their body to make a living.

In the context of a different case, that of Michel-Anne Drouart, the child of poor stocking-weavers, the author Vacherie explicitly comments on the fact that children with ambiguous genitals from more privileged social backgrounds were typically not accessible for the surgeon's scrutinizing gaze: "It is *pretended* that, that at *Lyons, Rue Merciere* there exists actually an Hermaphrodite truly perfect in both Sexes, but that by the care of the Parents, who are wealthy Merchants, and who will not permit an authentic Verification thereof, for the Satisfaction of the Public, the Reality … must remain undecided" (14; emphasis in original). Eighteenth-century surgeons' writings on "hermaphrodites" show how, as Anne McClintock argues, the "triangulated theme" of race, gender, and class came into existence "*in and through* relation to each other" (4; emphasis in original). Imperial subjects and socially and economically disadvantaged European individuals were increasingly juxtaposed in discussions of nonnormative sexualities. The sexuality of the laboring class, especially of its women, became suspect in a context of increasing industrialization made possible by imperialism.[22] In this respect, the fact that the Angolan was exhibited in the same space, Covent Garden, where the epitome of "working women"—prostitutes—advertised their services is significant. Both cater to the "satisfaction of the public" (Vacherie 14) in a voyeuristic consumer culture that connected the medical sphere to the publishing world and the imperial realm.

Parsons's stated goal in juxtaposing the Angolan and the domestic "hermaphrodite" in his discussion of Douglas's illustration was to prove that the Angolan had "nothing but what is common to every Woman" (140). However, the reason why the domestic subject was displayed in the first place were her ambiguous genitalia that aligned her with "hermaphroditism." At the same time that this comparison strove to preclude any debate about the Angolan's sex, it actually reified both subjects' association with "hermaphroditism." The illustration depicts, amid the Angolan's abundant curly hair, a genital structure that bears more resemblance to a penis than a clitoris. The result is a tension between the textual and the visual elements in

Parsons's treatise. While the text vehemently denies the conjecture that the clitoris might be a penis, the image suggests this possibility. Parsons was not the only physician who used Douglas's illustration. William Cheselden also reproduced it in four editions of his *Anatomy* (1722-41). He did so, however, to prove the exact opposite of Parsons (Fontes da Costa 136), namely that the Angolan displayed a perfect mixture of both sexes. "Hermaphrodites" were not an ontological reality but an epistemological creation by individual physicians in a specific context.

Domestic Drouart

Despite Parsons's attempt to establish "epistemological certainty" (Braunschneider 526) regarding "hermaphrodites," *Enquiry* is marked by an ambiguity that subsequent authors explore. Vacherie's *Account of the Famous Hermaphrodite*, published a decade later, in 1750, focuses on a domestic body, that of Michel-Anne Drouart, yet also resorts to a foreign subject when opposing his contemporaries' claims that there are no "hermaphrodites." In contrast to Parsons, whose goal in referencing the Angolan is to prove that all supposed "hermaphrodites" are only miscategorized women, Vacherie uses "a Negro *Hermophradite* [*sic*] *from Guinea*" (15; emphasis in original) to prove the existence of individuals who cannot be classified as either male or female. In the addenda included at the end of his account, Vacherie describes the Guinean as having ambiguous external genitalia. He acknowledges that "it is hard to decide, without such an Anatomical Research, as it is impossible during the Life of the Subject" (17), pointing at the necessity of an autopsy. At the same time, however, he concedes that even a postmortem dissection of the genitals would not provide all the answers:

> It can only be said, that was this the Case, the Difference would only be local, and confined to those Parts of Generation… the Ambiguity of its

> Sex is diffused over the whole Body of it, in a greater or lesser Degree … as make it doubtful to which this equivocal Being belongs. (17)

For Vacherie, markers of sexuality permeate the entire body, thereby thwarting efforts to establish epistemological certainty in a single anatomical structure.[23] If sex was everywhere, true human "hermaphrodites"—in the sense of individuals who possessed the reproductive potential of both sexes—were thinkable. In this respect, Vacherie argues that the Parisian "hermaphrodite"—Drouart—is more of a "hermaphrodite" than the Guinean, "whose *Penis* was though not of so perfect a Conformation, as that of the Parisian above described" (15; emphasis in original). According to him, "there is less wanting in this Subject [Drouart] towards this Perfection, than in any that are now known" (13–14). Vacherie's use of the term "perfection" actually refers to the *imperfect* formation of the genitals. Whereas Parsons highlighted imperfectly formed genitals as a sign of the "racial" other, the surgeon Vacherie was invested in proving that Europeans could also be "hermaphrodites" and that his work therefore had direct relevance for his contemporaries suffering from a condition that only he could diagnose and potentially cure. Of all the authors discussed in this book, Vacherie's professional and financial investment in the existence of "hermaphrodites" is the most pronounced. His broadside-style *Account* most visibly pursued the revenue potential for publications on human curiosities and, while doing so, strategically explored the ambiguous spaces in Parsons's *Enquiry*, thereby transforming readers into potential patients.

Nineteenth-Century Shifts

In the mid-eighteenth century, domestic and foreign "hermaphrodites" were examined side-by-side. In these comparative studies, the racial and sexual boundaries remained fluid despite the gradually consolidating two-sex model of sex and emerging theories of race. This conception of the body as a malleable entity was, however, disappearing at the beginning of the nineteenth century, as can be seen in Monorchis's 1801 publication on the Berlin case of Maria Dorothea Derrier. Whereas Parsons and Vacherie do not comment on the Angolan's or the Guinean's skin color, Monorchis explicitly does:

> The black hermaphrodite, who was shown later in London, was not at all different from the one just mentioned, except that the pitch-black color of his skin contributed more to his ugliness. The more clearly hermaphroditism manifests, the more the affected individual is dreadful and therefore unformed.
>
> [Der schwarze Hermaphrodite, den man späterhin zu London gezeigt, war von dem eben erwähnten gar nicht unterschieden, außer daß seine pechschwarze Gesichtsfarbe noch mehr zu seiner Hässlichkeit beitrug. Je mehr der Hermaphrodismus entschieden ist, je mehr muss auch das Individuum, bei welchem er sich vorfindet, ungeheuer, und folglich ungestaltet seyn. (15)]

Like his predecessors, Monorchis juxtaposes a domestic subject, Derrier, to a foreign subject of color. The foreign subject referenced here might be either the Guinean or the Angolan "hermaphrodite"; it could even be a different individual as the text does not provide any further identification. Tellingly, the subject is no longer referenced by geographical provenance but by skin color as the "black hermaphrodite." Skin color is emphasized by the adjective "pechschwarz" ("pitch black"), which is in turn aligned with "Hässlichkeit" ("ugliness"), projecting the subject into a space of absolute alterity. This shift points at the gradual consolidation of race as an essential biological marker.

In Monorchis's case history, Derrier is, however, not only compared to the Black "hermaphrodite"; the "earlier mentioned Drouart" ["eben erwähnten [Drouart]]," a French subject, is also invoked. Monorchis observes Drouart's "*un*verschämte Gesichtsbildung" ["outrageous facial formation"] (14; emphasis added). "Unverschämt," on the one hand, refers to the supposedly odd appearance of Drouart's face ("outrageous") and, on the other, implies a lack of shame—unver*schäm*t ("impudent"; emphasis added)—and thereby makes claims regarding its bearer's moral character. In this context, Derrier's face appears in stark contrast to Drouart's: "The formation of her [Derrier's] face does not have the imprint of disgust or repulsiveness that typically characterizes those of her kind; she has a rather pleasing appearance" ["Ihre [Derriers] Gesichtbildung hat nicht das Gepräge von Ekel oder Widrigkeit, was andere ihres Gleichen sonst gemeiniglich auszeichnet, sie ist vielmehr von einem gefälligen Ansehn"] (5). In addition to observing Derrier's agreeable face, Monorchis also implicitly opposes Derrier's "shameful blushing and unspoiled mores" ["Schamröthe und Unverdorbenheit der Sitten"] to Drouart's character, thereby ranking Derrier above both Drouart and the Black "hermaphrodite" in terms of appearance and morality.[24]

Monorchis argues that the appearance of the Black "hermaphrodite" is even less pleasing than that of the French subject, Drouart, yet what unites them in his opinion is that they are both "*un*gestaltet" and "*un*geheuer" (emphases added). The use of adjectives with the prefix "un-" is significant in this context. Rather than using the word "missgestaltet"—"malformed"—Monorchis coins the word "ungestaltet," which can be translated as "unformed." Drouart and the Black "hermaphrodite" both appear stuck in a stage of development that does not allow their physical formation to progress. "Ungeheuer" as an adjective means "dreadful"; as a noun it stands for "monster." Monorchis projects both Drouart and the Black "hermaphrodite" into the realm of alterity. In Monorchis's hierarchization of different peoples, Drouart, the French subject, occupies an intermediary space between the Berlin "hermaphrodite" Derrier and the nameless Black "hermaphrodite" exhibited in London.

Monorchis thereby positions Drouart as an example of French moral decline. In the European context, the French nation was frequently aligned with the excesses of its aristocracy, which were thought to cause effeminacy and the weakening of the entire body politic.[25] Because the German and

British bourgeoisie emulated fashionable French manners through their habits of consumption, France was considered to have a harmful effect on domestic vitality throughout Europe. Class anxieties were gendered and became translated into fears about shifting gender roles. Those fears led to the suspicion of the female body, which was translated into investigations into physiques that were considered nonstandard. These investigations, in turn, enabled physicians to strengthen their own professional and social standing. In Monorchis's satire of his contemporaries' infatuation with scientific oddities, French culture figures prominently, especially in the conclusion, which imagines a tipsy-turvy world where "Germany will be inundated by womanish division generals à la Xentrailles" ["Deutschland von weibischen Divisions-Generalen à la Xentrailles überschwemmt [wird]"] (16). In addition to being one of the few female freemasons in the eighteenth century, Madame de Xentrailles, the German-born Marie-Henriette Heiniken, disguised herself as a man and served as a soldier during the Napoleonic Wars. This cross-dressing leads to a questioning of gender roles that intersects with the perceived threat of French culture and politics overtaking not only individual German bodies but the body politic of the entire European continent ("Lady Freemasons" 191).

Madame Xentrailles is an ambivalent figure. On the one hand, she represents German apprehension of the feminizing effects of French culture while, on the other, she is masculinized by her depiction as a general. At the time that Monorchis was writing, people in German territories feared the effects of the French Revolutionary Wars (1796–1802) at home. A female war-faring figure like Madame de Xentrailles became a symbol of the existing social and political uncertainty and, therefore, generated the same fascination and anxieties as the "hermaphrodites" that the public eagerly viewed.[26] Monorchis argues that "nearly all hermaphrodites are merely girls, in whom the tools of their sex have developed too much and reach beyond the typical boundaries" ["fast alle Hermaphroditen nur Mädchen sind, bei welchen sich die Werkzeuge ihres Geschlechts zu sehr entwickelt haben und über die gewöhnlichen Gränzen erstrecken"] (7). Even though Monorchis posits that Derrier is female, the fear of the challenge that bodies such as Derrier's and Madame de Xentrailles's pose to sexual boundaries and gender norms surfaces in his pseudonym "Monorchis," referring to a man with a single testicle.

For Monorchis, the most vexing aspect about women with overdeveloped clitorises was their appearance on the European continent, more specifically, in Berlin:

> This phenomenon is all the more striking in our climes considering that the ancient and most reliable observations teach us that only in those areas that lie between the thirtieth degree latitude and the line [the equator], the genitals of women are larger than in other countries.
>
> [Diese Erscheinung ist unter unserm Himmelsstriche um so auffallender, als die uralten und zuverlässigsten Beobachtungen uns lehren, daß nur in jenen Gegenden, welche zwischen dem dreyßigsten Grade nördlicher Breite und der Linie liegen, die Geschlechtsteile der Weiber ausgedehnter sind, als in andern Ländern.] (5–6)

Monorchis subscribed to the theory that climate affected physical constitution. The "heat of the climate that slackens ... all fibers" ["Hitze des Klimas ... die alle Fiebern erschlafft"] (6) was seen as the cause of the "disorderly expansion of the clitoris and the nymphae" ["unordentliche Ausdehnung der Klitoris, und der Nymphen"] (6). The fact that a Berlin woman also presented with an elongated clitoris contributed to Monorchis's generalized feeling of unease, both in a medical and a political context. Derrier became the signifier of a world on the brink of chaos. Monorchis's anxiety about the future of his own territory, Berlin Brandenburg, surfaces several times in the introduction and the conclusion to his treatise. Fears of French invasion were not unfounded; Napoleon eventually marched into Berlin in 1806, five years after Monorchis had published his study. The Napoleonic Wars would lead to the reorganization of Europe with the

Congress of Vienna in 1815, which also set the stage for full-fledged colonialism. Colonial discourse would further blur the line between domestic and foreign subjects at the same time that it strove to consolidate it.

Monorchis's 1801 satire on the medical and popular infatuation with "hermaphrodites," of which he himself was a part, expresses the discomfort with a rapidly changing world: "Heaven protect us from a republic of hermaphrodites with masculine hearts and feminine minds" ["Dann behüte uns der Himmel vor einer Republik von Hermaphroditen mit Männerherzen und Weibersinn"] because then "there will be more of the bizarre, ridiculous, defective, evil in the world than there unfortunately already is!!! in addition to the realm of hermaphrodites" ["des Bizarren, den Lächerlichen, Schadhaften und Bösen in der Welt weit mehr werde, als leider!!! außer dem Reiche der Hermaphroditen, schon vorhanden ist"] (16). While the reference to gender and sexuality functions metaphorically in this description of a topsy-turvy world, it also has a literal dimension as it reveals a deep *angst* about a world in which everything is being rethought, including the prominence of men in the political and professional realm. What if those who hold a "Gebärmutter" (uterus)—which Monorchis abbreviates as "Bärmutter"—literally translatable as "mother of bears"—would rule the world? What would be the ramifications if more individuals from regions beyond Europe, like the African "hermaphrodite," entered the homeland and blurred those sexual and racial boundaries upon which the political and social status quo depended?

The eighteenth-century imagination of sexually ambiguous bodies as *terra incognita* crystallizes the confluence of anxieties regarding gender, race, ability, and class. At the same time that the social and professional status of medicine and in particular surgery rose, some of its practitioners such as Burghart and Monorchis adopted a satirical perspective toward it. The increasing prominence of surgery in the medical realm became the topic of various satires that existed alongside treatises publicizing the virtues of anatomical demonstration and surgical intervention. Next to the advertisement of the Angolan exhibit, which extolled the authority of three prominent anatomists and surgeons—Douglas, Freak, and Cheselden—the March 24, 1741 issue of the *London Daily Post and General Advertiser* included an announcement for Henry Fielding's play *The Mock-Doctor or the Dumb Lady Cur'd* (1732). This farce, an adaptation of Molière's *Le médecin malgré lui*, details the adventures of a British woodcutter who disguises himself as a French doctor named Ragou. The choice of the name "Ragou" represents contemporaries' ambivalence toward medicine's increasing focus on anatomical dissection that resembled the woodcutting practices of the protagonist. The fact that Fielding's play was performed at Covent-Garden, the same space where the Angolan was exhibited alongside prostitutes, illustrates the complex intersection of the medical profession with consumer culture. Both were complicit in the creation of liminal bodies as "hermaphrodites" in the eighteenth century and in the resulting erasure of their agency. Only in later centuries will these individuals reclaim their voice by responding to medical discourse with their embodied experience.

Notes

1 In this context, Malick W. Ghachem notes that "not a single major scholar of the French Revolution has produced important work on colonial history" (7). He also argues that Foucault "simplified the legal history of the Old Regime" (9) and thereby French colonial history.

2 On this point, see Kenneth Morgan: "Spanish depredation on Bristol-based shipping began before the outbreak of war, but the situation deteriorated between 1739 and 1740 when at least seventeen Bristol vessels were captured by Spanish privateers" (*Bristol* 18–19).

3 Some of the cited reasons for this decline are the lack of successors in prominent Bristol merchant families and the failure to industrially develop the Bristol hinterlands. On the role of Bristol in the Atlantic slave trade, also see Armitage and Braddick, Dresser, Morgan (*Bristol* and *Slavery*), and Sacks.

4 This location gradually became the center of London over the course of the eighteenth century, supplanting areas to the East. The status of Charing Cross as the city center was cemented in the early nineteenth century, when Trafalgar Square was built on

its site to memorialize Lord Nelson's 1805 victory over the French and Spanish in the Battle of Trafalgar.

5 For a discussion of the history of syphilis, see Merians, Reinarz, and Quétel. In fact, as Noelle Gallagher observes, in the eighteenth century, venereal diseases were often associated with the foreign, in particular "not those who remained completely outside the nation, but those who influenced or infiltrated it—those, in other words, who threatened to compromise the boundaries between foreigner and native" (115).

6 This exclamation was a version of the phrase "Mas, Mulier, Monachus [monk]; Mundi mirabile Monstrum!" (Neugebauer 258; also in Dreger, *Hermaphrodites* 214), which had been used to reference the discovery of female sex in a monk. The replacement of "monk" with "moor" testifies to imperial realities of the eighteenth century.

7 For an account of popular entertainment from the Elizabethan to the Victorian era, see Altick.

8 On this point, see Porter, "Consumption."

9 For a discussion of the female body in the context of eighteenth-century consumer culture, see Hilger, "The Feminine Performance" and "The 'Weibliche Geschlechte.'"

10 The original Latin reads *Systema naturæ per regna tria naturæ, secundum classes, ordines, genera, species, cum characteribus, differentiis, synonymis, locis.*

11 A discussion of the way that climate was thought to shape European national character can be found in Hilger, "Writing Back."

12 See Arnold for an account of the description of equatorial areas in the emerging field of tropical medicine.

13 On the topic of domesticity in the novel, see Armstrong and May.

14 Buffon's chapter "Variétés dans l'espèce humaine" [Varieties in the human species] from his *Histoire naturelle* (1749) was particularly influential in this respect because it was published with the king's imprimatur (Andrew Curran 118).

15 For centuries, travelogues had reported the presence of light-skinned Africans. While these individuals had been mythologized for centuries, in a manner similar to humans with variable sex characteristics, in the eighteenth century scientists sought to explain their origins. In 1744, four years after the exhibit of the Angolan, a four-year old "nègre blanc" was displayed in Paris. In his 1745 treatise *Vénus physique*, the French philosopher and mathematician Pierre Louis Moreau de Maupertius discussed this phenomenon. Like Parsons, Maupertius included the physical exam at the end of his text because he first refuted a more mythological explanatory model, the theory of preformation. Maupertius theorized that the birth of an albino could be understood in the context of monogenesis.

16 For an insightful account of the medicalization of Blackness in the Atlantic world, see Hogarth.

17 A 1779 London case of gender reassignment surgery is described by Warren.

18 "Fricatrices" and female masturbation from the seventeenth to the nineteenth centuries are examined in Braunschneider, Sharrock, and Traub.

19 On the issue of the internal hierarchization of European nations, see Hilger, *Gender* 107–32.

20 Douglas's illustration showed the London woman with both the labia closed and opened. The fact that Douglas's plate of the Angolan only depicted the opened labia led Parsons to produce an additional plate that showed them in their closed state, in analogy to Douglas's illustrations of the London woman: "As Dr Douglas's Plate only shews the Labia of the Parts of the Angolan woman opened, it was necessary that a Figure of the same should precede it with the Labia shut or closed; that the Reader might better understand … of which the following is the Explanation" (Parsons 155).

21 Discourses of gender and imperialism are closely intertwined in the foldout, which bears resemblance to a landscape with craters, hills, ridges, and forests that, in its mystery and opaqueness, calls for investigation and exploration.

22 See Clark for a discussion of the sexuality of the eighteenth-century laboring classes and gender roles.

23 See Schiebinger's *The Mind Has No Sex?* for eighteenth-century anatomists' view that sex permeated all anatomical structures.

24 The use of physical appearance—in particular that of the face—to describe an individual's character points at the increasing importance of physiognomy and its contribution to the development of scientific racism in the early nineteenth century (Schiebinger, *Nature's Body* xi). Physiognomy was revived from classical antiquity in the eighteenth century by Johann Kaspar Lavater. While esoteric at first, it was gradually appropriated by medicine and entered mainstream discourse. Like Monorchis, Lavater engages in a comparative analysis of people from different regions of the globe. In one of these analyses, he "points out that the negro of Angola and the Calmuck have facial angles below seventy degrees and that 'a further diminution soon loses all trace of resemblance to humanity' (495)" (Wechsler 107). See Percival, Warman, and Wechsler on Lavater's role in the revival of physiognomy in the eighteenth century.

25 For a discussion of German fears regarding the influence of French mores and manners, see Hilger, "The 'Weibliche Geschlechte.'"

26 For a discussion of the way female cross-dressed warriors figured in the literary imagination, see Hilger, *Gender*.

Conclusion

In Jeffrey Eugenides's 2002 novel, *Middlesex*, the protagonist Calliope Stephanides describes how a family friend, during a dinner-table conversation, discusses the "preformationists, with their roller-coaster names—Spallanzani, Swammerdam, Leeuwenhoek—[who] believed that all humankind had existed in miniature since Creation." (199). Dr. Philobosian, a physician, explains to the Stephanides family that eighteenth-century preformationists came to their conclusions after examining silkworms. Silkworms provide the narrative link between eighteenth-century preformationists and the Stephanides family, the members of which fled Asia Minor for the United States in the early twentieth century after having farmed silkworms for generations. Preformationists' inquiry into silkworms was embedded in eighteenth-century debates about reproduction and sexual development. In *Middlesex*, these two issues also stand at the center of the protagonist's identity quest in the early twenty-first century: Calliope Stephanides is intersex, born with 5-alpha-reductase deficiency, a recessive condition attributable to the fact that Calliope's grandparents were siblings. Raised as a girl, Calliope begins to question their identity during their teenage years. When, in search of answers for their unusual physique, Calliope visits the New York Public Library, they are struck by the sheer size of the dictionary located at the center of the reading room:

> I had never seen such a big dictionary before. The Webster's at the New York Public Library stood in the same relation to other dictionaries of my acquaintance as the Empire State Building did to other buildings. It was an ancient, medieval-looking thing, bound in brown leather that brought to mind a falconer's gauntlet. The pages were gilded like the Bible's. (430)

The dictionary's monumental size and its patina mark its authority. Its gilded pages eventually lead Calliope to the entry for "hermaphrodite," the term that overlaps yet is not completely synonymous with "intersex." The *Webster*'s entry allows Calliope to make sense of their physician's medical jargon and his plan to surgically normalize their genitals. Calliope's observation that "here was a book that contained the collected knowledge of the past" (431) highlights the central role played by reference works in the curation and dissemination of knowledge. Reference works fully assumed this privileged position during the Enlightenment, with the publication of the *Encyclopédie, ou Dictionnaire raisonné des sciences, des arts et des métiers* (1751–72). The *Webster*'s towering presence in twenty-first-century America mirrors the status of the monumental collection of knowledge spearheaded by Denis Diderot and Jean d'Alembert in mid-eighteenth-century Europe.

The conclusions of medical case histories on so-called "hermaphrodites" were incorporated into Enlightenment reference works such as the *Encyclopédie*. The *Encyclopédie* thereby further contributed to the dissemination and popularization of medical knowledge regarding gender and sexuality. The *Encyclopédie* (1751–66) and its sequel, the *Supplément à l'Encyclopédie* (1776–7), both contain an entry on the "hermaphrodite." The ontological construction of the "hermaphrodite" in these entries is a process that illustrates the tensions underlying not just the encyclopedic venture but the Enlightenment project at large. After summarizing the story of Hermaphroditus from Greek mythology, the author of the *Encyclopédie* entry, Louis de Jaucourt, concludes that there are no real-life "hermaphrodites"—humans with the capacity to function both as the male and the female in the reproductive process—because Enlightenment scientists can uncover whether the supposed "hermaphrodite" is, in fact, man or woman. At the same time that such conclusions establish an opposition between the "facts" of science and the "fiction" of mythology, they also expose the fact that the boundaries between these two realms were fluid. Like the case history, which was constructed with elements from both genres, encyclopedic entries are open-ended, necessitating the publication of further entries in eighteenth-century science's epistemological quest. The fact that the first volume of the *Supplément* appeared in 1776, a mere four years after the publication of the *Encyclopédie*'s last installment, illustrates this process. The *Supplément* was published by a different group of intellectuals (Marc-Michel Rey, Charles-Joseph Panckoucke, and Jean-Baptiste-René Robinet), who felt the need for corrections.[1] Over a six-year period, the editors bought and borrowed articles by a variety of authors from a wide range of countries and intellectual backgrounds, which were then summarized, paraphrased, and sometimes directly collated into the *Supplément*.

In the *Supplément*, the *Encyclopédie*'s central question—"But are there true hermaphrodites?"—is transformed into "But aren't there true *hermaphrodites*?" ["Mais n'y a-t-il pas de véritables *hermaphrodites*?"] (Haller 359; emphasis in original). By positioning itself with respect to the *Encyclopédie*'s outright denial of "hermaphrodites," this part of the *Supplément* article—authored by Albrecht von Haller, one of the scientists who was deeply enmeshed in the preformationist-epigenesist debate and who changed his position over the course of his career—reveals the epistemological doubt that is present between the lines of the *Encyclopédie*. Both the content and the form of the *Supplément* article foreground questions rather than provide answers. In comparison to the original, three-page *Encyclopédie* entry, the *Supplément* article has doubled in size. Not only has the entry expanded considerably, but it also occupies relatively more space in the *Supplément*, which—in contrast to the

Encyclopédie's seventeen volumes—consists of only four. In addition, while the *Encyclopédie* article was composed by a single writer, Jaucourt, the *Supplément* entry was penned by three authors (Albrecht von Haller, Hugues Maret, and an unnamed contributor) who, in turn, collated material from other writers into their parts of the entry. The collaborative aspect of this project further highlights the constructedness of the knowledge that scientists strove to present as objective and factual, as well as their own position in it.[2]

Encyclopedic entries and case histories construct the "hermaphrodite" as an object of study in the eighteenth century. Both are situated in the space where science and entertainment intersect, resulting in a highly voyeuristic, commodified, and therefore problematic form of entertainment science that was built on Europe's imperial ventures during this period. These ventures were predicated on the abjection of individuals according to race, class, ability, and sex and gender. Reading these case histories is disconcerting, painful, and triggering. Yet it is important to do so in order not only to understand the way in which eighteenth-century physicians viewed individuals they believed did not fit in the operative categories of their time but also to uncover the historical basis for present-day attempts to normalize bodies that are considered nonstandard. In order not to reify eighteenth-century beliefs about race, class, ability, and sex and gender, it is important to read these texts against the grain. This means not reading them as statements of facts but rather as claims that are deeply vested in their authors' position in eighteenth-century medicine and the commercialization of science. Using the tools of literary-critical analysis to read these case histories allows us to denaturalize their construction of the "hermaphrodite" and question the presentation of biological variation as a pathology.

Case histories, the premiere genre of medical discourse, illustrate the intersections between scientific and literary accounts of individual bodies. By undoing the science-literature dichotomy that it seeks to codify, this genre highlights the fact that medicine is not a science per se but an interpretive practice that draws on analytical methods from a variety of disciplines. The eighteenth century constitutes a transitional period as it is situated in-between the de facto interdisciplinarity that had reigned until the early modern period and the disciplinary specialization that would become institutionalized over the course of the nineteenth century. At the same time that eighteenth-century medical men disavowed their indebtedness to the humanistic realm, they drew on it when crafting their case histories. Faced with the shift from eighteenth-century case histories on living "hermaphrodites" to nineteenth-century microscopic exams of postmortem tissue and therefore pure materialism, physicians expressed concerns. Prominent Paris surgeon Sauveur François Morand's *Discours dans lequel on prouve qu'il est nécessaire au chirurgien d'être lettré* [Treatise in which it is proven that a surgeon needs to be lettered] (1743) registers the anxieties generated by this development, arguing for a type of medicine that is at least as humanistic as it is scientific.

Morand's ideal of the lettered surgeon resembles Friedrich Schiller's concept of the "Universalgelehrte" ["universal scholar"], which he presented in his inaugural lecture as a professor of history at the University of Jena in May 1789.[3] Addressed to his fellow historians and students, Schiller opposed the "Brotgelehrte" ["bread scholar"] to the "philosophische Kopf" ["philosophical head"] (5). Schiller, known as much for his contributions to German literature as for his historical writings, argued that the scholar who works primarily to earn an income, his bread, is interested in separating his discipline from all others so as to protect his academic territory and carefully circumscribe his tasks. By contrast, the philosophical head incarnates the Enlightenment ideal of the universal scholar whose goal is to connect his studies to different disciplines in an effort to insert them into the "wide whole of the world" ["große Ganze der Welt"] (7). Schiller reacted to the gradually increasing disciplinary specialization and highlighted the inadequacy of any type of epistemological endeavor that did not strive to understand the "connection between things" ["Zusammenhang der Dinge"] (7) by failing to embed discipline-specific knowledge into a broader context. Schiller's ideal of the philosophical head acknowledges the reality that, by the late eighteenth century, disciplinary boundaries had become jealously guarded by those working within their comforting confines. Schiller's reflections on scholarship and research were shaped profoundly by the disciplinary rift that he experienced in his own life. In addition to being a historian and playwright,[4] Schiller was also a physician; he, therefore, had to straddle the gap between medicine and literature carefully and strategically.[5]

The analysis of eighteenth-century case histories on "hermaphrodites" demonstrates the importance of interdisciplinary scholarship. Over the past few decades, the Health Humanities has established itself as the premiere field that enables interdisciplinary approaches to a variety of textual genres.[6] These approaches not only enable an understanding of the blurred boundaries between scientific and nonscientific texts but also denaturalize concepts of masculinity and femininity. By unsettling binary conceptions, interdisciplinary approaches are particularly productive for studies of corporeality and embodiment that explore the intersectionality of identities with respect to sex, gender, race, class, and ability. Questions of embodiment occupy a prominent place in the analysis of the medical discourse on "hermaphrodites," especially at a time when bodies were thought to be malleable. Even though the eighteenth-century medical men discussed in this book did not surgically reshape their subjects' bodies, they frequently alluded to the feasibility of such interventions.[7] The practice of surgically normalizing nonnormative bodies became common in the 1960s and was the extension of the Enlightenment's effort to organize the world into clearly demarcated categories. Twentieth-century surgeons followed in the footsteps of their eighteenth-century predecessors and became the enforcers of the regulatory law that strove to deny the body's ambiguity. The twentieth-century scalpel became an extension of the eighteenth-century pen, which had erased the embodied experience of the "hermaphrodite" from the pages of history.

Only in the late twentieth- and early twenty-first century did the authority of the scalpel begin to be questioned and, with it, the normative pronouncements of past and present medical discourse.[8] Published at the turn of the millennium, Jeffrey Eugenides's *Middlesex* is part of this context. Named after the muse of narrative poetry, the intersex protagonist Calliope writes their own story when they resist their parents' and physicians' decision to surgically normalize their genitals. Calliope does so by consulting the entry "hermaphrodite" in the *Webster's*. Rather than acquiescing to its description of nonstandard bodies as "freaks" or "monsters," Calliope realizes that their doctor's plans for surgery are part of a long-standing narrative regarding physical alterity. Eugenides positions his novel, the fictional autobiography of an intersex protagonist, as a response to the historical representation of nonbinary individuals as objects of medical discourse rather than as agents of their own destiny. That Eugenides features eighteenth-century theories about reproduction as a topic of conversation at the Stephanides dinner table attests to their significance for present-day notions of sex and gender.

While Eugenides's Pulitzer Prize-winning fictional intersex autobiography has been discussed extensively in scholarship, real-life accounts of intersex people have been met with less scholarly interest, as Katelyn Dykstra observes:

> While sociologists briefly reference these memoirs in their studies of the biomedicalization of intersex bodies, there are few in-depth studies of the texts themselves because literary scholars do not consider them as worthy of serious study. That intersex memoirs have, for the most part, not been examined in meaningful ways in literary studies speaks to both the invisibility of intersex in our society and the generic instability of the genre of the memoir, situated on the border between history and literature. (35)

The Health Humanities provide a productive context within which to analyze intersex life-writing, a genre that falls in-between the cracks of more traditional types of scholarship.[9] Discussing the intersex life writings published in the 2015 issue of the journal *Narrative Inquiry in Bioethics*, Dykstra shows how these writers respond to modern medical discourse. Their reference point becomes the medical chart, to which they oppose their own embodied experience of living with a body deemed nonstandard. The present-day medical chart is an institutionalized extension of the medical case history, which, as this book has shown, started to play an increasingly important role in the eighteenth century's ontological construction of the "hermaphrodite" as a category in medical discourse. Retracing these historical developments is therefore the first step on the path to recovering the subjectivity of those whose bodies question binaries relating not only to sex and gender but also to race, class, and ability. While there are no eighteenth-century writings *by* those liminal bodies, a close reading of the medical case histories *about* them traces their destabilization of normative discourse and, by doing so, uncovers their resistance to it. This resistance paved the way for later activist writing, which strove to recover the agency that medical discourse had taken from those whose bodies did not fit into neat classificatory schemes.

Notes

1 Kathleen Hardesty describes the complex publication history of the *Encyclopédie* and its relation to the *Supplément*.

2 For an extensive discussion of "hermaphrodite" entries in the *Encyclopédie* and the *Supplément*, see Hilger, "Orientation."

3 "Was heißt und zu welchem Ende studiert man Universalgeschichte?" [What does universal history mean and to what end does one study it?"]

4 For scholarship on Schiller as a historian and the connection to his literary production, in particular his historical tragedies, see, among others, Dann et al., Hoffmann et al., Kerry, Kimura, Prüfer, and Saranpa.

5 Schiller's medical training and his role as a physician have been garnering increasing critical attention during the past decade. See, for example, Engelhardt, Schäfer and Neuhausen, Sutermeister, Weiss, and Werner.

6 For a history of the Health Humanities, see Hilger, "Introduction." Also see DeTora and Hilger for the connection between the Health Humanities and embodiment studies. For a discussion of the intersection between the Health Humanities and eighteenth-century studies, see Hilger, "Medical Humanities."

7 There is one reported eighteenth-century case of surgery on a sexually ambiguous body. See Warren.

8 For twentieth- and twenty-first-century critiques of the medical management of intersex people, see Chase, Diamond (all), Griffiths (all), Hegarty (all), Karkazis, Kessler, Morland (all), Parens, Preves, and Bruce Wilson.

9 On this point, see Katelyn Dykstra and Shoshannah Bryn Jones Square's collection, *Intersex and the Health and Medical Humanities.*

WORKS CITED

Primary Texts

Burghart, D. Gottfried Heinrich. *Gründliche Nachricht an seinen Freund *** Von einem neuerlich gesehenen Hermaphroditen, Wobey zugleich etwas von der Medicinischen Mode erwähnet wird.* Breslau: Daniel Pietsch und Compagnie, 1763.

Champeaux, Claude. *Réflexions sur les Hermaphrodites relativement à Anne Grand-Jean, qualifiée telle dans un Mémoire de M. Vermeil, Avocat au parlement.* Avignon et Lyon: Claude Jacquenod, 1765.

Delius, Heinrich Friederich. "III. Nachricht von dem besondern Hermaphroditen Drouart." In *Fränkische Sammlungen von Anmerkungen aus der Naturlehre Arzneygelahrtheit Oekonomi und den damit verwandten Wissenschaften, einundvierzigtes* Stück. Nürnberg: Bei George Peter Monat, 1765, 398–405.

Des Essarts, Nicolas-Toussaint Le Moyne. *Procès fameux extraits de l'"Essai sur l'histoire générale des tribunaux tant anciens que modernes,"contenant les anecdotes piquantes, et les jugements fameux des tribunaux de tous les temps et de toutes les nations, par M. Des Essarts, avocat, member de plusieurs academies, secrétaire ordinaire de Monsieur, frère du roi.* Paris: Chez l'Auteur, 1788.

Ferrein, Antoine. *Mémoire sur le véritable sexe de ceux qu'on appelle hermaphrodites. Mémoires de l'Académie Royale des Sciences.* Paris: Imprimerie Royale, 1767, 330–9.

Fores, Samuel. *Man-Midwifery Dissected; or, the Obstetric Family Instructor for the Use of Both Sexes. Containing a Display of the Management of Every Class of Labour by Men and Boy Mid-Wives; also of Their Cunning, Indecent and Cruel Practices. Instructions to Husbands How to Counteract Them. A Plan for the Complete Instruction of Women Who Possess Promising Talents, in Order to Supersede Malepractice. Various Arguments and Quotations, Proving, that Man-Midwifery Is a Personal, Domestic and a National Evil.* London: Wellcome Library, 1793.

Haller, Albrecht von, Hugues Maret, and anonymous. "Hermaphrodite." In *Supplément à l'Encyclopédie, ou dictionnaire raisonné des sciences, des arts et des métiers. Par une société de gens de lettres*, vol. 3. Amsterdam: Chez MM Rey, 1777, 359–60.

Hoin, Jean Jacques Louis. *Nouvelle Description de l'Hermaphrodite Drouart, tel qu'on le voit à Dijon en août 1761.* Dijon: Veuve Coignard, 1761.

Hufeland, Christoph Wilhelm. "Beschreibung und Abbildung eines zu Berlin beobachteten Hermaphroditen." *Journal der practischen Arzneikunde und Wundarzneykunst* 12.3 (1801): 170–2.

Jaucourt, Louis de. "Hermaphrodite, Sub. & Adj. (Anat.)." In *Encyclopédie, ou dictionnaire raisonné des sciences, des arts et des métiers, etc*, edited by Robert Morrissey, vol. 6.

University of Chicago: ARTFL Encyclopédie Project (Spring 2013 Edition), 165–7. http://encyclopedie.uchicago.edu/ (accessed April 5, 2024).

Maret, M. "Description d'un hermaphrodite." *Mémoires de l'Académie de Dijon*, 1774, 157–69.

Martens, Franz Heinrich. *Beschreibung und Abbildung einer sonderbaren Misstaltung der männlichen Geschlechtsheile von Maria Dorothea Derrier aus Berlin nebst den Meinungen von Stark, Hufeland, Mursinna, monorchis über diese Person: Mit zwey colorierten Kupfern*. Leipzig: Baumgärtnerische Buchhandlung, 1802.

Mayer. "Description Anatomique d'un Hermaphrodite connu tour-à-tour sous les noms de Marie Dorothée Derier et Charles Durgé; par M. le professeur Mayer, de Bonn." *Gazette Médicale de Paris* 1836: 609–11.

Mayer. "Description of An Hermaphrodite, Known Under the Respective Names of 'Marie Dorothée Derrier' and 'Charles Dürge.' – by Professor Mayer, of Bonn." *The Lancet* 27.685 (1836): 140–2.

Mertrud, Antoine (and Jacques-Fabien Gautier d'Agoty). *Hermaphrodite, Dissertation au sujet de la fameuse hermaphrodite qui a paru aux yeux du public depuis environ trois mois, faite par le sieur Mertrud*. Paris: Berryer, 1749.

Monorchis, F. F. *Von dem neuangekommenen Hermaphroditen in der Charité zu Berlin im Jahre 1801 und von Zwittern überhaupt*. Berlin: Johann Wilhelm Schmidt, 1801.

Morand, Sauveur-François. "Description d'un hermaphrodite, que l'on voyait à Paris en 1749." In *Garçon et filles hermaphrodites vus et dessinés d'après nature par un des plus célèbres artistes et gravés avec tout le soin possible pour l'utilité des studieux*, edited by Jean-Michel Moreau. Paris: n.p., 1773. (Reprint of the original published *in Mémoires de l'Académie Royale des Sciences de Paris*, 1750).

Morand, Sauveur-François. *Discours dans lequel on prouve qu'il est nécessaire au chirurgien d'être lettré*. Paris: Charles Osmont, 1743.

Moreau, Jean-Michel (le Jeune). *Garçon et Fille hermaphrodites vus et dessinés d'après nature par un des plus célèbres artistes et gravés avec tout le soin possible pour l'utilité des studieux*. Paris: n.p., 1773.

Mursinna, Christian Ludwig. "Von einer besondern Naturbegebenheit." *Journal für die Chirurgie, Arzneikunde und Geburtshülfe* 1 (1801): 555–9.

Parsons, James. *A Mechanical and Critical Enquiry into the Nature of Hermaphrodites*. London: Printed for J. Walthoe, 1741.

Simon, Edouard-Thomas. *L'hermaphrodite ou Lettre de Grandjean a Françoise Lambert, sa femme*. Grenoble: n.p., 1765.

Stark, Johann Christian. "Kurze Beschreibung eines sogenannen Hermaphroditen oder Zwitters." *Neues Archiv für die Geburtshülfe, Frauenzimmer- und neugebohrner Kinderkrankheiten* 2.3 (1801): 538–56.

Vacherie, M. *An Account of the Famous Hermaphrodite, or, Parisian Boy-Girl, Aged Sixteen, Named Michael-Anne Drouart*. London: Samuel Johnson, 1750.

Vermeil, F. M. *Mémoire pour Anne Grandjean, connu sous le nom de Jean-Baptiste Grandjean, Accusé & Appelant. Contre Monsieur le Procureur general, accusateur et intimé*. Paris: Louis Cellot, 1765.

Secondary Literature

Accord Alliance. "Disorders of Sex Development." http://www.accordalliance.org/glossary/disorder-of-sex-development (accessed March 14, 2022).
Accord Alliance. "Homepage." http://www.accordalliance.org. (accessed March 18, 2020).
Aderibigbe, Moses Oludare. "A Philosophical Appraisal of the Concept of Common Origin and the Question of Racism." *Open Journal of Philosophy* 5 (2015): 25–30.
Altick, Richard. *The Shows of London*. Boston: Belknap, 1978.
Aravamudan, Srinivas. *Tropicopolitans: Colonialism and Agency, 1688–1804*. Durham: Duke UP, 1999.
Ariès, Philippe, and Georges Duby. *Histoire de la vie privée*, 5 vols. Paris: Seuil, 1985–1987.
Armitage, David, and Michael J. Braddick, eds. *The British Atlantic World, 1500–1800*. New York: Palgrave Macmillan, 2002.
Armstrong, Nancy. *Desire and Domestic Fiction: A Political History of the Novel*. Oxford: Oxford UP, 1987.
Arnold, David. *Warm Climates and Western Medicine: The Emergence of Tropical Medicine, 1500–1900*. Amsterdam: Rodopi, 1996.
Aulie, Richard. "Caspar Friedrich Wolff and His 'Theoria Generationis,' 1759." *Journal of the History of Medicine and Allied Sciences* 16.2 (April 1961): 124–44.
Behrens, Rudolf, and Carsten Zelle. *Der ärztliche Fallbericht: Epistemische Grundlagen und textuelle Strukturen dargestellter Beobachtung*. Wiesbaden: Harrassowitz, 2012.
Bell, Matthew. "The Economics of Authorship in Eighteenth-Century Germany and Britain." *Publications of the English Goethe Society* 86.3 (2017): 172–82.
Belling, Catherine. "Hypochondriac Hermeneutics: Medicine and the Anxiety of Interpretation." *Literature and Medicine* 25.2 (Fall 2006): 376–401.
Bettcher, Talia Mae. "Intersexuality, Transgender and Transsexuality." In *The Oxford Handbook of Feminist Theory*, edited by Lisa Disch and Mary Hawkesworth. Oxford: Oxford UP, 2016. 407–27.
Blackwood, Ashleigh, and Helen Williams. "Writing Doctors and Writing Health in the Long Eighteenth Century." *Journal for Eighteenth-Century Studies* 46.1 (March 2023): 3–20.
Bleker, Johanna, and Volker Hess, eds. *Die Charité: Geschichte(n) eines Krankenhauses*. Berlin: Akademieverlag, 2010.
Blum, Carol. *Strength in Numbers: Population, Reproduction, and Power in Eighteenth-Century France*. Baltimore: Johns Hopkins UP, 2002.
Bohm, Arnd. "Aufklärung, Inc.: Publishing in Eighteenth-Century Germany." *Eighteenth-Century Studies* 36.2 (Winter 2003): 286–88.
Bonner, Thomas Neville. *Becoming a Physician: Medical Education in Britain, France, Germany, and the United States, 1750–1945*. New York: Oxford UP, 1995.
Braunschneider, Theresa. "The Macroclitoride, the Tribade and the Woman: Configuring Gender and Sexuality in English Anatomical Discourse." *Textual Practice* 13.3 (1999): 509–32.

Brockliss, Laurence, and Colin Jones. *The Medical World of Early Modern France*. Oxford: Oxford UP/Clarendon Press, 1997.
Brown, Michael. *Emotions and Surgery in Britain, 1792–1912*. Cambridge: Cambridge UP, 2002.
Brown, Michael. *Performing Medicine: Medical Culture and Identity in Provincial England, c. 1760–1850*. Manchester: Manchester UP, 2014.
Buckley, Jenifer. *Gender, Pregnancy, and Power in Eighteenth-Century Literature: The Maternal Imagination*. London: Palgrave Macmillan, 2017.
Buffon, George-Louis Leclerc (Comte de). *Histoire naturelle, générale et particulière, avec la Description du Cabinet du Roi*. Paris: Imprimerie nationale, 1749–1804.
Calhoun, Craig, ed. *Habermas and the Public Sphere*. Cambridge: MIT, 1992.
Carey, Daniel, and Lynn Festa, eds. *The Postcolonial Enlightenment: Eighteenth-Century Colonialism and Postcolonial Theory*. Oxford: Oxford UP, 2009.
Chambers, Tod. *The Fiction of Bioethics: Cases as Literary Texts*. New York: Routledge, 1999.
Charles, Guy-Uriel, and Luis Fuentes-Rohwer. "Habermas, the Public Sphere, and the Creation of a Racial Counterpublic." *Michigan Journal of Race and Law* 21 (2015): 1–21.
Chase, Cheryl, and Martha Coventry, eds. Special Issue on Intersexuality. *Chrysalis: The Journal of Transgressive Gender Identities* 2.5 (Fall/Winter 1997).
Cheselden, William. *The Anatomy of the Human Body*. London: N. Cliff, D. Jackson, and W. Innys, 1713.
Cheselden, William. *The Anatomy of the Human Body*. London: Bowyer, 1741.
Chico, Tita. *The Experimental Imagination: Literary Knowledge and Science in the British Enlightenment*. Stanford: Stanford UP, 2018.
Chico, Tita. "Minute Particulars: Microscopy and Eighteenth-Century Narrative." *Mosaic* 39.2 (June 1, 2006): 143–61.
Clare, Eli. *Brilliant Imperfection: Grappling with Cure*. Durham: Duke UP, 2017.
Clark, Anna. *The Struggle for the Breeches: Gender and the Making of the British Working Class*. Berkeley: U of California P, 1997.
Class, Monika. "Introduction: Medical Case Histories as Genre: New Approaches." *Literature and Medicine* 32.1 (Spring 2014): vii–xvi.
Cobb, Matthew. *The Egg and Sperm Race: The Seventeenth-Century Scientists Who Unravelled the Secrets of Sex, Life, and Growth*. London: Simon and Schuster, 2006.
Cody, Lisa Forman. *Birthing the Nation: Sex, Science, and the Conception of Eighteenth-Century Britons*. Oxford: Oxford UP, 2005.
Collins, Patricia Hill. "Some Group Matters: Intersectionality, Situated Standpoints, and Black Feminist Thought." In *A Companion to African-American Philosophy*, edited by Tommy L. Lott and John P. Pittman. Malden: Blackwell, 2003, 205–29.
Curran, Andrew S. *The Anatomy of Blackness: Science and Slavery in an Age of Enlightenment*. Baltimore: Johns Hopkins UP, 2011.
Curran, Mark. *The French Book Trade in Enlightenment Europe I: Selling Enlightenment*. London: Bloomsbury, 2018.
Dahlberg, Lincoln. "The Habermasian Public Sphere: Taking Difference Seriously." *Theory and Society* 34.2 (April 2005): 111–36.

Dann, Otto, Norbert Oellers, and Ernst Osterkamp, eds. *Schiller als Historiker.* Stuttgart: Metzler, 1995.
Darnton, Robert. *The Business of Enlightenment: A Publishing History of the Encyclopédie, 1775–1800*. Boston: Belknap Press, 1987.
Darnton, Robert. *The Literary Underground of the Ancien Régime*. Cambridge: Harvard UP, 1982.
Darnton, Robert. "Reading, Writing, and Publishing in Eighteenth-Century France: A Case Study in the Sociology of Literature." *Daedalus* 100.1 (Winter 1971): 214–56.
Darnton, Robert, and Daniel Roche, ed. *Revolution in Print: The Press in France 1775–1800.* Berkeley: U of California P, 1989.
Daston, Lorraine, and Katharine Park. "The Hermaphrodite and the Orders of Nature: Sexual Ambiguity in Early Modern France." *Gays and Lesbians Quarterly* 1.4 (1995): 419–38.
Daston, Lorraine, and Katharine Park. *Wonders and the Order of Nature, 1150–1750.* New York: Zone Books, 2001.
Dean-Jones, Leslie. "Menstrual Bleeding according to the Hippocratics and Aristotle." *Transactions of the American Philological Association* 119 (1989): 177–92.
De Bellaigue, Christina. *Educating Women – Schooling and Identity in England and France, 1800–1867.* Oxford: Oxford UP, 2007.
DeJean, Joan. *Libertine Strategies: Freedom and the Novel in Seventeenth-Century France.* Columbus: Ohio State UP, 1981.
DeJean, Joan. "The Politics of Pornography." In *The Invention of Pornography: Obscenity and the Origins of Modernity, 1500–1800*, edited by Lynn Hunt. New York: Zone Books, 1996, 109–23.
DeJean, Joan. *The Reinvention of Obscenity: Sex, Lies, and Tabloids in Early Modern France.* Chicago: U of Chicago P, 2002.
De Renzi, Silvia. "Women and Medicine." In *The Healing Arts: Health, Disease and Society in Europe*, edited by Peter Elmer. Manchester: Open University, 2004, 196–227.
De Souza, Igor H. "Elenx de Cespedes: Indeterminate Genders in the Spanish Inquisition." In *Trans Historical: Gender Plurality Before the Modern*, edited by Greta LaFleur, Masha Raskolnikov, and Anna Klosowska. Ithaca, NY: Cornell UP, 2021, 42–67.
DeTora, Lisa M., and Stephanie M. Hilger. "Introduction." In *Bodies in Transition in the Health Humanities: Representations of Corporeality*, edited by Lisa M. DeTora and Stephanie M. Hilger. London: Routledge, 2020, 1–8.
Deutsch, Helen. *Resemblance & Disgrace: Alexander Pope and the Deformation of Culture.* Boston: Harvard UP, 1996.
Deutsch, Helen, and Felicity Nussbaum, eds. *"Defects": Engendering the Modern Body.* Ann Arbor: U of Michigan P, 2000.
DeVun, Leah. "The Jesus Hermaphrodite: Science and Sex Difference in Premodern Europe." *Journal of the History of Ideas* (April 2008): 193–218.
DeVun, Leah. *The Shape of Sex: Nonbinary Gender from Genesis to the Renaissance*: New York: Columbia UP, 2021.
DeVun, Leah, and Zeb Tortorici. " 'Trans*Historicities': A Roundtable Discussion." *Transgender Studies Quarterly Quarterly* 5.4 (November 2018): 658–85.

Diamond, Milton. “Pediatric Management of Ambiguous and Traumatized Genitalia.” *The Journal of Urology* 162 (1999): 1020–8.

Diamond, Milton. “Sex, Gender, and Identity Over the Years: A Changing Perspective.” *Child and Adolescent Psychiatric Clinics of North America: Sex and Gender* 13 (2004): 591–607.

Dirks-Schuster, Whitney. “Print Culture and the Monstrous Hermaphrodite in Early Modern England” (unpublished paper).

Douglas, Aileen. *Uneasy Sensations: Smollett and the Body*. Chicago: U of Chicago P, 1995.

Dreger, Allice Domurat. *Hermaphrodites and the Medical Invention of Sex*. Cambridge: Harvard UP, 1998.

Dreger, Allice Domurat. *Intersex in the Age of Ethics*. Hagerstown: University Publishing Group, 1999.

Dresser, Madge. *Slavery Obscured: The Social History of the Slave Trade in an English Provincial Port*. London: Bloomsbury, 2001.

Düwell, Susanne, and Nicolas Pethes, eds. *Fall—Fallgeschichte—Fallstudie: Theorie und Geschichte einer Wissensform*. Frankfurt: Campus Verlag, 2014.

Dykstra, Katelyn. “Charting Intersex: Intersex Life-Writing and the Medical Record.” In *Bodies in Transition in the Health Humanities: Representations of Corporeality*, edited by Lisa M. DeTora and Stephanie M. Hilger. London: Routledge, 2020, 35–44.

Dykstra, Katelyn, and Shoshannah Bryn Jones Square, eds. *Intersex and the Health and Medical Humanities*. London: Bloomsbury, 2022.

Eger, Elizabeth, Charlotte Grant, Clíona Ó Gallchoir, and Penny Warburton, eds. *Women, Writing and the Public Sphere, 1700–1830*. Cambridge: Cambridge UP, 2001.

Einhäupl, Karl Max. *300 Jahre Charité—im Spiegel ihrer Institute*. Berlin: Walter de Gruyter, 2010.

Engelhardt, Dietrich von. “Schillers Leben mit der Krankheit im Kontext der Pathologie und Therapie um 1800.” In *Schillers Natur: Leben, Denken, und literarisches Schaffen*, edited by Georg Braungart and Bernhard Greiner. Hamburg: Felix Meiner Verlag, 2005, 57–73.

Epstein, Julia. “Either/Or – Neither/Both: Sexual Ambiguity and the Ideology of Gender.” *Genders* 7 (Spring 1990): 99–142.

Epstein, Julia. “Historiography, Diagnosis and Poetics.” *Literature and Medicine* 11.1 (1992): 23–44.

Eugenides, Jeffrey. *Middlesex*. New York: Picador, 2002.

Farr, Jason S. *Novel Bodies: Disability and Sexuality in Eighteenth-Century British Literature*. Lewisburg: Bucknell UP, 2019.

Fausto-Sterling, Anne. *Sexing the Body: Gender Politics and the Construction of Sexuality*. New York: Basic Books, 2000.

Fissell, Mary. “The Marketplace of Print.” In *Medicine and the Market in England and its Colonies, c.1450–c.1850*, edited by Mark S. R. Jenner and Patrick Wallis. Houndmills: Palgrave, 2007, 108–32.

Fontes da Costa, Palmira. “ ‘Mediating Sexual Difference’: The Medical Understanding of Human Hermaphrodites in Eighteenth-Century England.” *Cultural Approaches to the History of Medicine: Mediating Medicine in Early Modern and Modern Europe*, edited by Willem de Blécourt and Cornelie Usborne. Houndmills: Palgrave Macmillan, 2004, 127–47.

Foucault, Michel. *Les anormaux: Cours au Collège de France (1974–1975)*. Paris: Gallimard/Seuil, 1999, 62–8.

Foucault, Michel. *Birth of the Clinic: An Archeology of Medical Perception*. New York: Vintage Books, 1994.

Foucault, Michel. *Herculine Barbin dite Alexina B*. Paris: Gallimard, 1978.

Foucault, Michel. *Naissance de la Clinique: Une archéologie du regard medical*. Paris: Presses universitaires de France, 1963.

Frank, Marcie. *The Novel Stage: Narrative Form from the Restoration to Jane Austen*. Lewisburg: Bucknell UP, 2020.

Fraser, Nancy. "Rethinking the Public Sphere: A Contribution to the Critique of Actually Existing Democracy." *Social Text* 25/26 (1990): 56–80.

Ftacek, Julia, "Jonathan Swift and the Transgender Classroom." *Journal for Eighteenth-Century Studies* 43.3 (2020): 303–14.

Furdell, Elizabeth. *Publishing and Medicine in Early Modern England*. Rochester: U of Rochester P, 2007.

Garland-Thomson, Rosemarie. *Extraordinary Bodies: Figuring Physical Disability in American Literature and Culture*. New York: Columbia UP, 1996.

Gelfand, Toby. *Professionalizing Modern Medicine: Paris Surgeons and Medical Science and Institutions in the Eighteenth Century*. London: Greenwood Press, 1980.

Gestrich, Andreas. "The Public Sphere and the Habermas Debate." *German History* 24.3 (July 2006): 413–30.

Geyer-Kordesch, Johanna. "Court Physician and State Regulation in Eighteenth-Century Prussia: The Emergence of Medical Science and the Demystification of the Body." In *Medicine at the Courts of Europe, 1500–1837*, edited by Vivian Nutton. London: Routledge, 1990, 155–82.

Geyer-Kordesch, Johanna. "German Medical Education in the Eighteenth Century: The Prussian Context and Its Influence." In *William Hunter and the Eighteenth-Century Medical World*, edited by W. F. Bynum and Roy Porter. Cambridge: Cambridge UP, 1985, 177–205.

Ghachem, Malick W. "Montesquieu in the Caribbean: The Colonial Enlightenment between *Code Noir* and *Code Civil*." In *Postmodernism and the Enlightenment*, edited by Daniel Gordon. New York: Routledge, 2001, 7–30.

Gilbert, Ruth. *Early Modern Hermaphrodites: Sex and Other Stories*. Houndmills: Palgrave Macmillan, 2002.

Goodman, Dena. *The Republic of Letters: A Cultural History of the French Enlightenment*. Ithaca: Cornell UP, 1994.

Goulemot, Jean-Marie. *Ces livres qu'on ne lit que d'une main: Lecture et lecteurs de livres pornographiques au XVIIIième siècle*. Aix-en-Provence: Alinéa, 1991.

Graille, Patrick. *Les hermaphrodites au xvii and xviiiième siècles*. Paris: Les Belles Lettres, 2001.

Griffiths, David Andrew. "Diagnosing Sex: Intersex Surgery and 'Sex Change' in Britain 1930–1955." *Sexualities* 21.3 (2018): 476–95.

Griffiths, David Andrew. "Shifting Syndromes: Sex Chromosome Variations and Intersex Classifications." *Social Studies of Science* 48.1 (2018): 125–48.

Guerrini, Anita. "Scots in London Medicine in the Early Eighteenth Century." In *Scots in London in the Eighteenth Century*, edited by Stana Nenadic. Lewisburg: Bucknell UP, 2010, 165–85.

Gurlt, Ernst. "Mursinna, Christian Ludwig." *Allgemeine Deutsche Biographie* 23 (1886): 81–4.

Habermas, Jürgen. *The Structural Transformation of the Public Sphere: An Inquiry into a Category of Bourgeois Society*. Trans. Thomas Burger. Cambridge: MIT Press, 1998.

Habermas, Jürgen. *Strukturwandel der Öffentlichkeit: Untersuchungen zu einer Kategorie der bürgerlichen Gesellschaft*. Darmstadt: Hermann Luchterhand Verlag, 1962.

Hacke, Daniela. *Women, Sex and Marriage in Early Modern Venice*. London: Routledge, 2017.

Hannaford, Ivan. *Race: The History of an Idea in the West*. Baltimore: Johns Hopkins UP, 1996.

Hardesty, Kathleen. *The Supplément to the Encyclopédie*. The Hague: Martinus Nijhoff, 1977.

Harrison, Mark. *Climates and Constitutions: Health, Race, Environment and British Imperialism in India 1600–1850*. Oxford: Oxford UP, 1999.

Harvey, Karen. *Reading Sex in the Eighteenth Century: Bodies and Gender in English Erotic Culture*. Cambridge: Cambridge UP, 2005.

Hegarty, P. "The Psychology of People with Variable Sex Characteristics/Intersex." *Current Opinion in Psychology* 49 (February 2023): n.p.

Hegarty, P., Prandelli, M., Lundberg, T., Liao, L.-M., Creighton, S., and Roen, K. "Drawing the Line between Essential and Non-Essential Interventions on Intersex Characteristics with European Healthcare Professionals." *Review of General Psychology* 25 (2021): 101–14.

Hegarty, P., and Smith, A. "Public Understanding of Intersex: An Update on Recent Findings." *International Journal of Impotence Research* 35 (2023): 72–7.

Hilger, Stephanie. *Gender and Genre: German Women Write the French Revolution*. Newark: U of Delaware P, 2014.

Hilger, Stephanie. "Introduction: Bridging the Divide between Literature and Medicine." In *New Directions in Literature and Medicine Studies*, edited by Stephanie Hilger. London: Palgrave Macmillan, 2017, 1–12.

Hilger, Stephanie. "Medical Humanities and the Eighteenth Century." *Goethe Yearbook* 28 (2021): 301–6.

Hilger, Stephanie. "Orientation and Supplementation: Locating the 'Hermaphrodite' in the *Encyclopédie*." *Goethe Yearbook* 22 (July 2015): 169–87.

Hoffmann, Michael. *Habermas's Public Sphere: A Critique*. Vancouver: Fairleigh Dickinson UP, 2017.

Hoffmann, Michael, Jörn Rüsen, and Mirjam Springer, eds. *Schiller und die Geschichte*. München: Wilhelm Fink, 2006.

Hogarth, Rana. *Medicalizing Blackness: Making Racial Difference in the Atlantic World*. Chapel Hill: U of North Carolina P, 2017.

Hohendahl, Peter Uwe. *The Institution of Criticism*. Ithaca: Cornell UP, 1982.
Holmes, Morgan. ed. *Critical Intersex*. Farnham: Ashgate, 2009.
Holmes, Morgan. *Intersex: A Perilous Difference*. Selinsgrove: Susquehanna UP, 2008.
Horsman, Reginald. *Race and Manifest Destiny: The Origins of Racial Anglo-Saxonism*. Harvard: Harvard UP, 1981.
Houston, R. A. *Literacy in Early Modern Europe: Culture and Education 1500–1800*. London: Longman, 2002.
Hull, Isabel. *Sexuality, State, and Civil Society in Germany, 1700–1815*. Ithaca: Cornell UP, 1996.
Hunt, Lynn, ed. *The Invention of Pornography: Obscenity and the Origins of Modernity, 1500–1800*. New York: Zone Books, 1996.
Intersex Society of North America. "What is Intersex?" http://www.isna.org/faq/what_is_intersex (accessed March 14, 2022).
Jacob, Margaret C. "The Materialist World of Pornography." In *The Invention of Pornography: Obscenity and the Origins of Modernity, 1500–1800*, edited by Lynn Hunt. New York: Zone Books, 1996, 157–202.
Jaeckel, Gerhart. *Die Charité: Die Geschichte des berühmtesten deutschen Krankenhauses*. Bayreuth: Hestia, 1963.
Jefcoate, Graham. "Am falschen Ort? German Printers and Booksellers in 18th Century London." In *Lire l'Autre dans l'Europe des Lumières*, edited by Andréa Gagnoud and Thomas Bremer. Montpellier: Presses Universitaires de la Méditerranée, 2007, 35–47.
Karkazis, Katrina. *Fixing Sex: Intersex, Medical Authority, and Lived Experience*. Durham: Duke UP, 2008.
Kaul, Suvir. "Provincials and Tropicopolitans: Eighteenth-Century Literary Studies and the Unmaking of 'Great Britain.'" *Diaspora* 9.3 (2000): 421–37.
Kavanagh, Declan. *Effeminate Years: Literature, Politics, and Aesthetics in Mid-Eighteenth-Century Britain*. Lewisburg: Bucknell UP, 2017.
Kelleher, Paul. *Making Love: Sentiment and Sexuality in Eighteenth-Century British Literature*. Lewisburg: Bucknell UP, 2015.
Keller, Eve. "'That Sublimest Juyce in Our Body': Bloodletting and Ideas of the Individual in Early Modern England." *Philological Quarterly* 86.1 (2007): 97–122.
Kerry, Paul, ed. *Friedrich Schiller: Playwright, Poet, Philosopher, Historian*. Oxford: Peter Lang, 2007.
Kessler, Suzanne. *Lessons from the Intersexed*. New Brunswick: Rutgers UP, 1998.
Kimura, Naoji. "Schillers 'Universalgeschichte,' ein idealistisches Programm?" In *Universalitätsanspruch und partikulare Wirklichkeiten: Natur- und Geisteswissenschaften im Dialog*, edited by Naoji Kimura and Karin Moser v. Filseck. Würzburg: Königshausen und Neumann, 2007, 93–106.
Klein, Ula Lukszo. *Sapphic Crossings: Cross-Dressing Women in Eighteenth-Century British Literature*. Charlottesville: U of Virginia P, 2021.
Kowaleski-Wallace, Elizabeth. *Consuming Subjects: Women, Shopping, and Business in the Eighteenth Century*. New York: Columbia UP, 1997.

Kronick, David. *A History of Scientific and Technical Periodicals: The Origins and Development of the Scientific and Medical Press, 1665–1799*. Lanham: Scarecrow Press, 1972.

Kronick, David. "Medical 'Publishing Societies' in Eighteenth-Century Britain." *Bulletin of the Medical Library Association* 82.3 (July 1994): 277–82.

"Lady Freemasons." *Masonic Review* 63.1 (February 1885): 190–2.

LaFleur, Greta. *The Natural History of Sexuality in Early America*. Baltimore: Johns Hopkins UP, 2018.

Landes, Joan. *Women and the Public Sphere in the Age of the French Revolution*. Ithaca: Cornell UP, 1988.

Laqueur, Thomas. *Making Sex: Body and Gender from the Greeks to Freud*. Cambridge: Harvard UP, 1990.

Lawrence, Susan C. "Anatomy and Address: Creating Medical Gentlemen in Eighteenth-Century London." *The History of Medical Education in Britain*, edited by Vivian Nutton and Roy Porter. Amsterdam: Rodopi, 1995, 199–228.

Lewes, Darby. "Utopian Sexual Landscapes: An Annotated Checklist of British Somatopias." *Utopian Studies* 7.2 (1996): 167–95.

Lindemann, Mary. "The Discourses of Practitioners in Eighteenth-Century France and Germany." In *The Cambridge World History of Medical Ethics*, edited by Robert Baker and Laurence McCullough. Cambridge: Cambridge UP, 2012, 391–8.

Lindemann, Mary. "Professionals? Sisters? Rivals? Midwives in Braunschweig, 1750–1800." In *The Art of Midwifery: Early Modern Midwives in Europe*, edited by Hilary Marland. London: Routledge, 1993, 176–91.

Linnaeus, Carl. *Systema naturæ, sive regna tria naturæ systematice proposita per classes, ordines, genera, & species*. Leiden: Haak, 1735.

Linton, Anne E. *Unmaking Sex: The Gender Outlaws of Nineteenth-Century France*. Cambridge: Cambridge UP, 2022, 1–18.

London Daily Post and General Advertiser January 15, 1741 (Issue 1944). 17–18th Century Burney Collection Newspapers.

London Daily Post and General Advertiser February 6, 1741 (Issue 1963). 17–18th Century Burney Collection Newspapers.

London Daily Post and General Advertiser March 24, 1741 (Issue 2002). 17–18th Century Burney Collection Newspapers.

London Daily Post and General Advertiser May 2, 1741 (Issue 2036). 17–18th Century Burney Collection Newspapers.

Long, Kathleen Perry. *Hermaphrodites in Renaissance Europe*. Aldershot: Ashgate, 2006.

Lubey, Kathleen. *Excitable Imaginations: Eroticism and Reading in Britain, 1660–1760*. Lewisburg: Bucknell UP, 2014.

MacLean, Ian. *Renaissance Notion of Woman: A Study in the Fortunes of Scholasticism and Medical Science in European Intellectual Life*. Cambridge: Cambridge UP, 1980.

Mak, Geertje. *Doubting Sex: Inscriptions, Bodies, and Selves in Nineteenth-Century Hermaphrodite Case Histories*. Manchester: Manchester UP, 2012.

Malatino, Hilary. *Queer Embodiment: Monstrosity, Medical Violence, and Intersex Experience*. Lincoln: U of Nebraska P, 2019.

Mallipeddi, Ramesh. *Spectacular Suffering: Witnessing Slavery in the Eighteenth-Century British Atlantic*. Charlottesville: U of Virginia P, 2016.

Manheim, Ernst. *Aufklärung und öffentliche Meinung: Studien zur Soziologie der Öffentlichkeit im 18. Jahrhundert*. Stuttgart—Bad Cannstatt: Frommann-Holzboog, 1979.

Manion, Jen. *Female Husbands: A Trans History*. Cambridge: Cambridge UP, 2020.

Mann, Jenny. "How to Look at a Hermaphrodite in Early Modern England." *Studies in English Literature, 1500–1900* 46.1 (2006): 67–91.

Marcus, Steven. *The Other Victorians: A Study of Sexuality and Pornography in Mid-Nineteenth-Century England*. New York: Basic Books, 1974.

Marguillier, Auguste. *Un poète troyen au xviiie siècle: Edouard-Thomas Simon dit Simon de Troyes*. Troyes: Dufour-Bouquot, 1890.

Marland, Hilary, ed. *The Art of Midwifery: Early Modern Midwives in Europe*. London: Routledge, 1993.

May, Leila Silvana. "The Strong-Arming of Desire: A Reconsideration of Nancy Armstrong's *Desire and Domestic Fiction*." *English Literary History* 68.1 (Spring 2001): 267–85.

McCarthy, John, Stephanie Hilger, Nicholas Saul, and Heather Sullivan, eds. *The Early History of Embodied Cognition from 1740 to 1920: The "Lebenskraft" Debate and Radical Reality in German Science, Music, and Literature*. Amsterdam: Rodopi, 2015.

McClintock, Anne. *Imperial Leather: Race, Gender, and Sexuality in the Colonial Contest*. London: Routledge, 1995.

McClive, Cathy. *Menstruation and Procreation in Early Modern France*. London: Routledge, 2016.

McGuire, James. "La représentation du corps hermaphroditique dans les planches de l'*Encyclopédie*." *Recherches sur Diderot et sur L'Encyclopédie* 11 (1991): 109–29.

McInnis, Brian. "Haller, Unzer, and Science as Process." In *Lebenskraft and Radical Reality: Body, Mind, Soul, and Agency in German Thought, Music, and Literature* edited by John McCarthy, Stephanie Hilger, Nicholas Saul, and Heather Sullivan. Amsterdam: Rodopi, 2015, 89–112.

McLaren, Angus. "The Pleasures of Procreation: Traditional and Biomedical Theories of Conception." In *William Hunter and the Eighteenth-Century Medical World*, edited by W. F. Bynum and Roy Porter. Cambridge: Cambridge UP, 1985, 323–41.

McTavish, Lianne. *Childbirth and the Display of Authority in Early Modern France*. Aldershot: Ashgate, 2005.

Meehan, Johanna, ed. *Feminists Read Habermas: Gendering the Subject of Discourse*. New York: Routledge, 1995.

Merians, Linda Evi. *The Secret Malady: Veneral Disease in Eighteenth-Century Britain and France*. Lexington: UP of Kentucky, 1997.

Mitchell, David, and Sharon Snyder. *Narrative Prosthesis: Disability and the Dependencies of Discourse*. Ann Arbor: Michigan UP, 2001.

Mol, Annemarie. *The Body Multiple: Ontology in Medical Practice*. Durham: Duke UP, 2003.

Morgan, Clifford Naunton. "Surgery and Surgeons in 18th-Century London." *Annals of the Royal College of Surgeons of England* 42.1 (1968): 1–37.

Morgan, Kenneth. *Bristol and the Atlantic Trade in the Eighteenth Century.* Cambridge: Cambridge UP, 1993.

Morgan, Kenneth. *Slavery and the British Empire: From Africa to America.* Oxford: Oxford UP, 2007.

Morland, Iain. "Intersex Surgery between the Gaze and The Subject." *Transgender Studies Quarterly* 9.2 (May 2022): 160–71.

Morland, Iain, editor. Special issue on "Intersex and After." *Gays and Lesbians Quarterly* 15.2 (2009).

Müller, Johannes Peter. *Bildungsgeschichte der Genitalien aus anatomischen Untersuchungen an Embryoen des Menschen und der Thiere.* Düsseldorf: Arnz, 1830.

Murray, Jacqueline. "One Flesh, Two Sexes, Three Genders?" In *Gender and Christianity in Medieval Europe*, edited by Lisa M. Bitel and Felice Lifshitz. Philadelphia: U of Pennsylvania P, 2013, 34–51.

Neugebauer, Franz von. "Hermaphrodism in the Daily Practice of Medicine: Being Information upon Hermaphrodism Indispensable to the Practitioner." *British Gynecological Journal* 19 (1903): 226–63.

Nussbaum, Felicity A. *The Limits of the Human: Fictions of Anomaly, Race and Gender in the Long Eighteenth Century.* Cambridge: Cambridge UP, 2003.

Nussbaum, Felicity A. *Torrid Zones: Maternity, Sexuality, and Empire in Eighteenth-Century English Narratives.* Baltimore: Johns Hopkins UP, 1995.

Orland, Barbara. "White Blood and Red Milk: Analogical Reasoning in Medical Practice and Experimental Physiology (1560–1730)." In *Blood, Sweat, and Tears: The Formation of Early Modern Medicine: Physiology*, edited by M. Horstmanshoff, Helen King, and Claus Zittel. Leiden: Brill, 2012, 443–80.

Outram, Dorinda. *The Enlightenment.* Cambridge: Cambridge UP, 2005.

Parens, Erik, ed. *Surgically Shaping Children: Technology, Ethics, and the Pursuit of Normality.* Baltimore: Johns Hopkins UP, 2006.

Park, Katharine, and Robert A. Nye. "Destiny Is Anatomy." Review *of Thomas Laqueur, Making Sex: Body and Gender from the Greeks to Freud. New Republic* February 18, 1991, 53–7.

Paster, Gail Kern. *The Body Embarrassed: Drama and the Discipline of Shame in Early Modern England.* Ithaca: Cornell UP, 1993.

Percival, Melissa. "Introduction." In *Physiognomy in Profile: Lavater's Impact on European Culture*, edited by Melissa Percival and Graeme Tytler. Newark: U of Delaware P, 2005, 15–24.

Pethes, Nicolas. "Telling Cases: Writing against Genre in Medicine and Literature." *Literature and Medicine* 32.1 (Spring 2014): 24–45.

Pfeifer, Klaus. *Medizin der Goethezeit: Christoph Wilhelm Hufeland und die Heilkunst des 18. Jahrhunderts.* Köln and Weimar: Böhlau, 2000.

Pinto-Correia, Clara. *The Ovary of Eve: Egg and Sperm and Preformation.* Chicago: U of Chicago P, 1997.

Pomata, Gianna. "Menstruating Men: Similarity and Difference of the Sexes in Early Modern Medicine." In *Generation and Degeneration: Tropes of Reproduction in Literature and History from Antiquity to Early Modern Europe*, edited by Valeria Finucci and Kevin Brownlee. Durham: Duke UP, 2001, 109–52.

Pomata, Gianna. "Sharing Cases: The Observations in Early Modern Medicine." *Early Science and Medicine* 15.3 (2010): 193–236.

Poovey, Mary. *A History of the Modern Fact: Problems of Knowledge in the Sciences of Wealth and Society*. Chicago: U of Chicago P, 1998.

Porter, Roy. "Consumption: Disease of the Consumer Society?" In *Consumption and the World of Goods*, edited by John Brewer and Roy Porter. London: Routledge, 1993, 58–84.

Porter, Roy. *The Greatest Benefit to Mankind: A Medical History of Humanity*. New York: Norton, 1997.

Pott, Sandra. "Literatur und Medizin im Jahrhundert: von der erneuerten Fortschrittskritik bis zum 'Medical Writing.'" *Gesnerus* 63 (2006): 127–43.

Pranghofer, Sebastian. "Changing Views on Generation: Images of the Unborn." In *The Secrets of Generation: Reproduction in the Long Eighteenth Century*, edited by Raymond Stephanson and Darren Wagner. Toronto: U of Toronto P, 2015, 167–94.

Preves, Sharon. *Intersex and Identity: The Contested Self*. New Brunswick: Rutgers UP, 2003.

Prüfer, Thomas. *Die Bildung der Geschichte: Friedrich Schiller und die Anfänge der modernen Geschichtswissenschaft*. Köln: Böhlau, 2002.

Quétel, Claude. *History of Syphilis*. Baltimore: Johns Hopkins UP, 1992.

Raven, James. *Publishing Business in Eighteenth-Century England*. Woodbridge: Boydell Press, 2014.

Read, Sara. "'Thy Righteousness Is but a Menstrual Clout': Sanitary Practices and Prejudice in Early Modern England." *Early Modern Women* 3 (2008): 1–25.

Reinarz, Jonathan. *A Medical History of Skin: Scratching the Surface*. London: Pickering and Chatto, 2013.

Richardson, Samuel. *Pamela; or, Virtue Rewarded*. London: Penguin, 1980.

Risse, Guenter. "Framing Gynecology in Edinburgh: The Perplexing Nature of Women's Bodies." In *New Medical Challenges during the Scottish Enlightenment*, edited by Guenter B. Risse. Amsterdam: Rodopi, 2005, 269–310.

Rivers, Isabel. *Books and their Readers in Eighteenth-Century England*. Leicester: Leicester UP, 1982.

Robilliard, Gabrielle. *Tending Mothers and the Fruits of the Womb: The Work of the Midwife in the Early Modern German City*. Stuttgart: Franz Steiner Verlag, 2017.

Roe, Shirley. *Matter, Life, and Generation: Eighteenth-Century Embryology and the Haller-Wolff Debate*. Cambridge: Cambridge UP, 1981.

Rolker, Christof. "Der Hermaphrodit und seine Frau: Körper, Sexualität und Geschlecht im Spätmittelalter." *Historische Zeitschrift* 297 (2013): 593–620.

Ronsil, Georges Arnaud de. "Dissertation sur les hermaphrodites." In *Mémoires de chirurgie, avec quelques remarques historiques sur l'état de la medicine et de la chirurgie en France et en Angleterre*, edited by Georges Arnaud de Ronsil. Paris: Dessain, 1768, 245–396.

Rubin, David. *Intersex Matters: Biomedical Embodiment, Gender Regulation, and Transnational Activism*. Albany: SUNY Press, 2017.

Runge, Laura L., and Pat Rogers, eds. *Producing the Eighteenth-Century Book: Writers and Publishers in England, 1650–1800*. Newark: U of Delaware P, 2009.

Sacks, David Harris. *The Widening Gate: Bristol and the Atlantic Economy, 1450–1700*. Berkeley: U of California P, 1993.

Saisselin, Rémy. *The Literary Enterprise in Eighteenth-Century France*. Detroit: Wayne State UP, 1979.

Salvaggio, Ruth. *Enlightened Absences: Neoclassical Configurations of the Feminine*. Urbana: U of Illinois P, 1988.

Samuels, Ellen. *Fantasies of Identification: Disability, Gender, Race*. New York: NYU Press, 2014.

Sangmeister, Dirk, and Martin Mulsow. *Deutsche Pornographie in der Aufklärung*. Göttingen: Wallstein, 2018.

Saranpa, Kathy. *Schiller's Wallenstein, Maria Stuart, and Die Jungfrau von Orleans: The Critical Legacy*. Rochester: Camden House, 2002.

Schäfer, D., and K. A. Neuhausen. "Schiller und die Medizingeschichte." *Sudhoffs Archiv* 98 (2014): 76–90.

Schiebinger, Londa. "Human Experimentation in the Eighteenth Century: Natural Boundaries and Valid Testing." In *The Moral Authority of Nature*, edited by Lorraine Daston and Fernando Vida. Chicago: U of Chicago P, 2004, 384–408.

Schiebinger, Londa. *The Mind Has No Sex?: Women in the Origins of Modern Science*. Cambridge: Harvard UP, 1989.

Schiebinger, Londa. *Nature's Body: Gender in the Making of Modern Science*. New Brunswick: Rutgers UP, 2013.

Schiebinger, Londa. *Plants and Empire: Colonial Bioprospecting in the Atlantic World*. Boston: Harvard UP, 2007.

Schiebinger, Londa. *Secret Cures of Slaves: People, Plants, and Medicine in the Eighteenth-Century Atlantic World*. Stanford: Stanford UP, 2004.

Schiller, Friedrich. "*Was heißt und zu welchem Ende studiert man Universalgeschichte?: Eine akademische Antrittsrede.*" Jena: In der akademischen Buchhandlung, 1789.

Schochow, Maximilian. *Die Ordnung der Hermaphroditen-Geschlechter: Eine Genealogie des Geschlechtsbegriffs*. Berlin: Akademie Verlag, 2009.

Schuller, Kyla, and Jules Gill-Peterson, "Introduction: Race, the State and the Malleable Body." *Social Text* 38.2 (June 2020): 1–17.

Sennett, Richard. *The Fall of Public Man*. New York: Knopf, 1976.

Sharrock, Cath. "Hermaphroditism; or, 'the Erection of a New Doctrine': Theories of Female Sexuality in Eighteenth-Century England." *Paragraph* 17.1 (1994): 38–48.

shuster, stef. *Trans Medicine: The Emergence and Practice of Treating Gender*. New York: NYU Press, 2021.

Siebers, Tobin. *Disability Theory*. Ann Arbor: U of Michigan P, 2008.

Smith, Courtney Weiss. *Empiricist Devotions: Science, Religion, and Politics in Early Eighteenth-Century England*. Charlottesville: U of Virginia P, 2016.

Smith, Lisa Wynne. "The Body Embarrassed? Rethinking the Leaky Male Body in Eighteenth-Century England and France." *Gender and History* 23.1 (April 2011): 26–46.

Smith, Lisa Wynne. "An Unusual Case of Menstruation in Eighteenth-Century England." http://sloaneletters.com/unusual-case-of-menstruation/ (accessed April 9, 2024).

Snow, C. P. *The Two Cultures and the Scientific Revolution*. London: Cambridge UP, 1959.

Soyer, François. *Ambiguous Gender in Early Modern Spain and Portugal*. Leiden: Brill, 2012.

Spary, E. C. "Health and Medicine in the Enlightenment." In *Oxford Handbook of the History of Medicine*, edited by Mark Jackson. Oxford: Oxford UP, 2011. 82–99.

Spary, E. C. *Utopia's Garden: French Natural History from Old Regime to Revolution*. Chicago: U of Chicago P, 2000.

Spencer-Hall, Alicia, and Blake Gutt. *Trans and Genderqueer Subjects in Medieval Hagiography*. Amsterdam: Amsterdam UP, 2021.

Spivak, Gayatri Chakravorty. "Can the Subaltern Speak?" In *Colonial Discourse and Postcolonial Theory: A Reader*, edited by Patrick Williams and Laura Chrisman. London: Routledge, 1994.

Stephanson, Raymond, and Darren N. Wagner. "Introduction." In *The Secrets of Generation: Reproduction in the Long Eighteenth Century*, edited by Raymond Stephanson and Darren N. Wagner. Toronto: U of Toronto P, 2015, 3–33.

Sterne, Laurence. *The Life and Opinions of Tristram Shandy, Gentleman*. London, 1759–67.

Stolberg, Michael. "Menstruation and Sexual Difference in Early Modern Medicine." In *Menstruation: A Cultural History*, edited by Andrew Shail and Gillian Howie. Houndmills: Palgrave Macmillan, 2005, 90–101.

Stolberg, Michael. "A Woman Down to Her Bones: The Anatomy of Sexual Difference in the Sixteenth and Seventeenth Centuries." *Isis* 94.2 (June 2003): 274–99.

Stoler, Ann Laura. *Race and the Education of Desire: Foucault's History of Sexuality and the Colonial Order of Things*. Durham: Duke UP, 1995.

Susen, Simon. "Critical Notes on Habermas's Theory of the Public Sphere." *Sociological Analysis* 5.1 (2011): 37–62.

Sussman, Charlotte. *Consuming Anxieties: Consumer Protest, Gender, and British Slavery, 1713–1833*. Stanford: Stanford UP, 2000.

Sutermeister, Hans. *Schiller als Arzt: Ein Beitrag zur Geschichte der psychosomatischen Forschung*. Bern: Haupt, 1955.

Systma, Sharon, ed. *Ethics and Intersex*. Dordrecht: Springer, 2006.

Thomas, Samuel. "Early Modern Midwifery: Splitting the Profession, Connecting the History." *Journal of Social History* 43.1 (2009): 115–38.

Thompson, Courtney E. "Questions of Genre: Picturing the Hermaphrodite in Eighteenth-Century France and England." *Eighteenth-Century Studies* 49.3 (Spring 2016): 391–413.

Thompson, Helen. *Fictional Matter: Empiricism, Corpuscles, and the Novel*. Philadelphia: U of Pennsylvania P, 2017.

Tougaw, Jason Daniel. *Strange Cases: The Medical Case History and the British Novel*. New York: Routledge, 2006.
Toulalan, Sarah. *Imagining Sex: Pornography and Bodies in Seventeenth-Century England*. Oxford: Oxford UP, 2007.
Toulalan, Sarah "'Unfit for Generation': Body Size and Reproduction." In *The Secrets of Generation: Reproduction in the Long Eighteenth Century*, edited by Raymond Stephanson and Darren Wagner. Toronto: U of Toronto P, 2015, 299–318.
Towler, Jean, and Joan Bramall. *Midwives in History and Society*. London: Croom Helm, 1986.
Traub, Valerie. "The Psychomorphology of the Clitoris." *Gays and Lesbians Quarterly* 2 (1995): 81–113.
Tuttle, Leslie. *Conceiving the Old Regime: Pronatalism and the Politics of Reproduction in Early Modern France*. New York: Oxford UP, 2010.
Van Horn Melton, James. *Absolutism and the Eighteenth-Century Origins of Compulsory Schooling in Prussia and Austria*. Cambridge: Cambridge UP, 2002.
Vicente, Marta. *Debating Sex and Gender in Eighteenth-Century Spain*. Cambridge: Cambridge UP, 2017.
Wahrman, Dror. *The Making of the Modern Self: Identity and Culture in Eighteenth-Century England*. New Haven: Yale UP, 2006.
Warman, Caroline. "What's Behind a Face? Lavater and the Anatomists." In *Physiognomy in Profile: Lavater's Impact on European Culture*, edited by Melissa Percival and Graeme Tytler. Newark: U of Delaware P, 2005, 94–108.
Warren, Carol A. B. "Gender Reassignment Surgery in the Eighteenth Century: A Case Study." *Sexualities* 17.7 (2014): 872–84.
Watt, Ian. *The Rise of the Novel: Studies in Defoe, Richardson, and Fielding*. Berkeley: U of California P, 1957.
Wechsler, Judith. "Lavater, Stereotype, and Prejudice." In *The Faces of Physiognomy: Interdisciplinary Approaches to Johann Caspar Lavater*, edited by Ellis Shookman. Columbia: Camden House, 1993, 104–25.
Weiss, Johannes. "Dichter und Denker: Friedrich Schiller und die Medizin." *Zeitschrift für Gastroenterologie* 52.3 (April 2014): 264.
Werner, Bernd. *Der Arzt Friedrich Schiller, oder, Wie die Medizin den Dichter formte*. Würzburg: Königshausen und Neumann, 2012.
Wheeler, Roxann. *The Complexion of Race: Categories of Difference in Eighteenth-Century British Culture*. Philadelphia: U of Pennsylvania P, 2000.
Wiehe, Jarred. "No Penis? No Problem: Intersections of Queerness and Disability in Laurence Sterne's *The Life and Opinions of Tristram Shandy, Gentleman*." *The Eighteenth Century* 58.2 (Summer 2017): 177–93.
Wiesner-Hanks, Merry E. "The Midwives of South Germany and the Public/Private Dichotomy." In *The Art of Midwifery: Early Modern Midwives in Europe*, edited by Hilary Marland. London: Routledge, 1993, 77–94.
Wiesner-Hanks, Merry E. *Women and Gender in Early Modern Europe*. Cambridge: Cambridge UP, 2008.

Wilson, Adrian. *The Making of Man-Midwifery: Childbirth in England 1660–1770*. Cambridge: Harvard UP, 1995.

Wilson, Bruce E., and W. G. Reiner. "Management of Intersex: A Shifting Paradigm." *Journal of Clinical Ethics* 9.4 (1998): 360–9.

Winckel, Franz von. "Martens, Franz Heinrich." *Allgemeine Deutsche Biographie* 20 (1884): 460–1.

Wizemann, T. M., and M. L. Pardue, eds. "Exploring the Biological Contributions to Human Health: Does Sex Matter?" Institute of Medicine Committee on Understanding the Biology of Sex and Gender Differences. Washington: National Academies Press, 2001.

Wolff, Michelle, David A. Rubin, and Amanda Lock Swarr. "The Intersex Issue: An Introduction." *Transgender Studies Quarterly* 9.2 (May 2022): 143–59.

Woods, Robert, and Chris Galley. *Mrs Stone & Dr Smellie: Eighteenth-Century Midwives and their Patients*. Liverpool: Liverpool UP, 2015.

INDEX

www.ingramcontent.com/pod-product-compliance
Ingram Content Group UK Ltd.
Pitfield, Milton Keynes, MK11 3LW, UK
UKHW020818290926
15470UKWH00003B/1225

9 781350 374928